COLLEC-TIVE BIOLO-GIES

Duke University Press   *Durham and London*   2021

COLLEC-TIVE

Healing Social Ills through Sexual Health Research in Mexico

BIOLO-GIES

EMILY A. WENTZELL

Project editor: Annie Lubinsky
Designed by Courtney Leigh Richardson and typeset in
Futura and Minion Pro by Westchester Publishing Services

Library of Congress Cataloging-in-Publication Data
Names: Wentzell, Emily A., [date] author.
Title: Collective biologies : healing social ills through sexual
health research in Mexico / Emily A. Wentzell. Description:
Durham : Duke University Press, 2021. | Includes
bibliographical references and index.
Identifiers: LCCN 2021012450 (print) |
LCCN 2021012451 (ebook)
ISBN 9781478013945 (hardcover)
ISBN 9781478014881 (paperback)
ISBN 9781478022176 (ebook)
Subjects: LCSH: Sexual health—Research—Socialaspects—
Mexico.|Medicine— Research—Socialaspects— Mexico. |
Collective behavior. | Group identity—Mexico. |
Individualism—United States. | BISAC: SOCIAL SCIENCE /
Anthropology / Cultural & Social | HISTORY / Latin
America/Mexico
Classification: LCC RA788 .W46 2021 (print) |
LCC RA788 (ebook) | DDC 613.90972—dc23
LC recordavailableathttps:// lccn.loc.gov/2021012450
LC ebookrec ordavailableathttps:// lccn.loc.gov/2021012451

Cover art: HPV virus. Courtesy Kateryna Kon/Science
Photo Library.

For Adam, Elliot, and Simon, who helped me understand
all that "living for others" stuff in chapter 4

CONTENTS

The pandemic has been a hell of a way to demonstrate this book's relevance.

This is a book about how people in a Mexican city destabilized by pre-pandemic economic and narcoviolence crises used a seemingly individual act—participating in medical research—to help others. They hoped to help by supporting science in the abstract, disinterested way imagined by Western medical ethics boards. Yet they also hoped men would directly benefit from the medical testing they received and that those benefits, in turn, would concretely enhance the embodied well-being of specific groups of others. The medical research participants I worked with understood themselves to be members of groups at different scales, from their families to the Mexican populace, whose collective, embodied futures were determined by all members' actions.

Here I call these bodies "collective biologies." My goal in doing that is to offer a way to theorize the nonindividual and embodied consequences of understanding oneself as part of a physically and socially interrelated group. It is obvious, though important, to note that everyone and everything is interrelated in a general sense. In this book I offer a way to theorize a particular kind of interrelationship. I analyze the ways that people's experiences of belonging in culturally recognizable groups, such as couples and congregations, shape their daily life actions and, in turn, influence collective well-being. I investigate how people's beliefs about the boundaries and contours of their own relationships with specific sets of others have embodied consequences for those others.

For the research participants I worked with, their memberships in these biosocial collectives were unremarkable, often implicit truths fundamental to daily life action. Theorizing them explicitly is my way of mapping the collective consequences of one ethnographic example of medical research. Further, it is an effort to provide a model for identifying how cultural ideologies of interrelatedness become embodied on greater-than-individual levels in other cases.

It is no accident that I felt called to try to understand this phenomenon while experiencing new forms of collective biology in my own life. In what could be considered intensive participant observation in embodied relatedness, I gave birth to two children between doing the fieldwork for this book and completing the final manuscript. These new beings depend on me and my husband to meet their needs and to engage in the joyful and exhausting social interactions that make us all people in cultures. I knew that kids need care. I naïvely did not realize how extensive the embodied consequences of providing it would be, from the surgical scar on my wrist that reflects the repetitive strain of childcare to the vastly different calculation of the consequences of my own risk taking that now shapes every new move I make. As members of a nuclear family in a society in which that unit is framed as the main locus of care, what happens in one of our bodies influences quite concretely what happens in the other three's bodies.

This became painfully clear when the COVID-19 pandemic struck. Our nuclear family became a bubble, and our interdependence and shared vulnerabilities, and the varying porosities of our collective bodily and social boundaries, became the main driver of every action we took. I had written about Mexican medical research participants trying to care for collectives amid crisis. Now I was consciously experiencing the state of "living for others" that people had told me about in our interviews not only through new parenthood, but also through my hopes that my own actions would protect the collectives to which I belonged from the harms of the COVID-19 pandemic. Like the research participants I interviewed in Mexico I hoped to be able to use my individual actions to effect change in several collectives, at multiple scales. For example, I hoped changes like teaching online would not only protect my family, but also contribute to the well-being of larger collectives such as my university community.

Yet being American during the pandemic, I have also experienced a cultural form that is opposite to my own hopes and those voiced by Mexican research participants: the refusal of collectivity. I live in Iowa, a midwestern U.S. state whose government refused to mandate masks even when we topped the global charts for COVID-19 positivity rates. Rejecting collectivities does not actually make the individualist fantasies fundamental to Anglo-American culture true or seal our bodies off from one another. We are all still interrelated, and your refusal to wear a mask can still sicken me and my children and their day care teachers and their families. But that refusal does preclude the kinds of care we can achieve when we understand ourselves to be members of specific groups affected by other group members' actions and bodies, and live accordingly.

While I feel them keenly as a new parent in a pandemic, this book's insights into enacting or refusing collective biologies extend past any moment or place. For instance, COVID-19 will eventually recede. Yet the ongoing pandemic of racism, disproportionately directing viral and other dangers to people of color, harms on a longer timeline. Many activists' efforts to redress this draw on ideologies of collective biology. Conversely, people's efforts to maintain and profit from institutionalized inequality might involve rejection of collectivity. Mask refusal as performance of Anglo-American individuality could fall into this category. Yet as American white supremacists' actions terrifyingly show, explicit efforts to maintain racialized inequalities can also represent perverse efforts to care for collective biologies to which people believe they belong. In the context I discuss in this book, people's understandings of themselves as Mexicans simultaneously make it feel possible for them to use individual medical research participation to aid the national populace, and reify the racial categories that naturalize gender inequality via *machismo*, and marginalization of Indigenous people and other Mexicans excluded from national narratives of progress through *mestizaje*.

I offer these examples of racialized collective biologies here both to highlight the relevance of the analytic of collective biologies in and beyond our current moment and to stress that this approach can be used to understand harms perpetrated in the name of promoting a collective's well-being. Collective biologies themselves are not inherently positive. Yet I hope that the analytic of collective biologies that this book presents can do some modest good.

In disciplines from anthropology to biology, we are developing new ways to understand the fundamental interrelatedness of the social and material aspects of the world, without reifying the ideas of a bedrock, essential "nature" that have created and justified so many forms of inequality. I hope that the concept of collective biologies will contribute to that work. I hope it will help us identify how the ideologies of collectivity present in particular places and times influence the embodied well-being of the people imagined to belong to those collectives. I hope it can be applied in a way that enables greater-than-individual bodies to be studied and understood in fields such as clinical research, which currently focuses on individuals even when investigating population-level phenomena. Finally, in a desire intensified by the desperation of the unmitigated pandemic and the exhaustion wrought by caring for those two new humans amid it, I hope that readers will be inspired by this book's examples of naming and caring for collectives to think in fresh ways through the collective consequences of their own actions, and to care for one another.

—October 15, 2020

ACKNOWLEDGMENTS

I am deeply grateful to the people who so graciously took the time to partici-pate in this research. The variety of ways you sought to help others, and your willingness to include interviews with an anthropologist among them, were truly inspirational. Your candor about life in challenging times, often along with humor and commiseration, touched me and made doing this work not only intellectually engaging but personally meaningful. Thank you.

This research would not have been possible without extremely generous support, assistance, and access from the leaders and staff of the Human Pap-illomavirus Infection in Men (HIM) study. Dr. Jorge Salmerón, head of the Cuernavaca arm of the HIM study and director of the Instituto Mexicano del Seguro Social's Epidemiology and Health Services Research Unit (the Unidad) in Cuernavaca, you have basically made my entire career possible through your willingness to provide access, space, help, and collaboration out of sheer enthusiasm for research and a desire to support colleagues in any field, at any career stage, from anywhere. I owe particular gratitude to Dr. Rossana Gonzalez Sosa, Licenciado Manuel Quiterio Trenado, and Enfermera (Nurse) Griselda Díaz for the intense and time-consuming logis-tical support you provided during the years of fieldwork for this research. All of the staff at the Unidad were kind and welcoming and offered crucial support for my work. I deeply value the friendships we have made over time, including, but not limited, to *mis queridas* Verónica Chavez, Lucinda Cruz, Vero Guadarrama, and Irma Villalba.

While it does not appear in this book, a week at the Tampa HIM site provided me with a key comparative understanding of the study. Thanks to Dr. Anna Giuliano, Principal Investigator of the HIM study, for supporting this project and hosting me in Tampa, and to the Tampa staff, especially Martha Abrahamsen and Christine Gage, for helping me do interviews there. These fieldwork trips were funded through my University of Iowa start-up and an Old Gold course release, which provided time for focused research. I owe my institution thanks for that support.

Some amazing friends in Cuernavaca have made it a second home rather than just a field site. Yvonne Flores, you are a fantastic friend, collaborator, spa/movie/restaurant buddy, and more. Your generosity in opening your home to me on so many research trips is staggering and greatly appreciated. Dulce Palomo and Ricardo Fragoso, you started out as roommates and will be friends for life. Thanks for making the non-work parts of my time in Mexico so much fun. Thanks also to Cathy Pepin and Christine Cretchley for hosting me one memorably delicious summer at the Casa Chocolate. Maria del Carmen Sánchez, I value your kindness and hope to see you and the extraordinarily good-humored Xoxocotla exercise group when it is possible to return to Mexico. Victor, I am grateful for the taxi rides but even more for your supportive presence and frequent help understanding life in Cuernavaca.

I am so lucky to have wonderful friends who, as fellow anthropologists, can help think through work and life at the same time. Becca Howes-Mischel, my steadfast writing group partner, thank you for *so* much feedback for so many years. Thanks also for managing somehow to be a cheerleader and a critical reader at the same time and for being a kind, insightful, and witty presence in my life, our field, and the world as a whole. Mikaela Rogozen-Soltar, thank you for always being there for me in the darkest and most absurd times, as well as the most delightful. You are brilliant, hilarious, generous in your listening and support, and a friend who makes me want to be better. I could not have made it through some hard times without you, and your friendship makes the good times so much better. Elana Buch, thank you for being a friend and colleague who listens, cares, and gets it. Talking to you about our work, teaching, and shared experiences of parenthood and life has made me much smarter and happier, and 100 percent less gaslighted. Jess Robbins, thank you for always reaching out, sharing, and listening. I don't think you realize that your resilience is contagious. Megan Styles, it's rare for someone so smart and insightful to also be so joyful. Thank you for being a positive presence in the world, as well as for your unfailing willingness to visit random tourist attractions. Graduate school friends Lizzy Falconi, Kelly Fayard, Kate Graber, and Karen Hébert, we don't get to see one another nearly enough, but just knowing that we periodically do makes me very happy. Megan Crowley-Matoka and Rebecca Seligman, our yearly meetups are brief but lovely moments of support and laughter that always renew my faith in our field. Eva Alcántara and Sarah Luna, my dissertation-era friends,

I rarely see you, but your work and selves constantly inspire me. Marcia Inhorn, I owe you a debt of gratitude for being my adviser, then collaborator, and always supporter and role model.

During the course of this project, so many more colleagues have generously provided feedback, support, help, and commiseration about research and career issues. Thanks to Rene Almeling, Margaret Beck, Raffaella Ferrero Camoletto, Cynthia Chou, Mariola Espinosa, Sherina Feliciano-Santos, Laurie Graham, Matt Hill, Iza Kavedzija, Meena Khandelwal, Susie Kilshaw, Ellen Lewin, Christine Labuski, Sarah Lamb, Katina Lillios, Caitrin Lynch, Anindita Majumdar, Sameena Mulla, Sarah Ono, Ted Powers, Erica Prussing, and Samantha Solimeo. Thanks also to Naomi Greyser and the participants in the Project on Rhetoric of Inquiry (POROI) seminar who provided helpful feedback on early ideas from this project. A big thanks to Shari Knight and Beverly Poduska, who provided daily support and kindness in the Anthropology Department office.

This book would not exist without the editorial staff at Duke University Press. Thanks to Ken Wissoker for helping me start this project, Gisela Fosado for seeing it through, and Alejandra Mejía for assistance along the way. Thanks also to the anonymous reviewers who were so generous with their time and ideas and whose feedback made this work much stronger.

I am lucky to have great friends in Iowa City who have made life during the long course of this project fun (in the good times) and bearable (in the bad). Thanks, Rachel Antonuccio-Jenkins, Ari Ariel, Erika Banks, Heather and Mark Bingham, Andy and Mary High, Lexy Ihrig, Lori Ihrig, and Yasmine Ramadan. Ali McDowell and Erin Daly, it feels like you have always been my friends (even though it's only been twenty-five years), and I'm so grateful that you always will be.

I owe special gratitude to some people who have helped make parenthood compatible with finishing this book and, frankly, sanity. Kathy Devine, Grace Schwarzendruber, and Felicia Wagner, you are outstanding birth professionals. I will never forget how the care and comfort you provided has enriched my life. Teachers and staff at Kids' Depot, you make our existence possible. Thanks for your joyful and trustworthy care for our kids and for teaching them so many Queen songs.

Finally, I am so grateful for my family. Lynn Puritz-Fine, thank you for raising me, moving to Iowa, becoming GG, and helping me get through grad school, tenure, childbirth, pandemic, and whatever next thing I know I can count on you for. Steve Wentzell, thank you for your unfailing support and for modeling talking to strangers. Who knew it would become my main career skill? Carole and John Yack, thank you for welcoming me into your family and always supporting my career.

Adam Yack, you are a wonderful husband, father, and human. Thank you for saying the sexiest words ever uttered by a man in a cis-het relationship: "We need to prioritize your career." Your belief in me, together with all the things you do to keep our lives going, made this book possible. I love you. Elliot, as a three-year-old you can't yet understand what sweetly calling your mom "My Little Anthropologist" and asking with real interest about my workday means, but you will. Simon, thanks for being so hilarious and adorably yourself at age one.

ONE

SEXUAL HEALTH RESEARCH, RELATIONSHIPS, AND SOCIAL CHANGE IN CUERNAVACA

Carjacking, Conversion, and HPV Research Participation

Arturo's path to becoming a medical research participant began when he was locked in a car trunk, praying for his life. The forty-five-year-old taxicab driver lived in the central Mexican city of Cuernavaca, a once-peaceful area stricken by an unprecedented wave of narcoviolence. One night, he was carjacked. Two men beat him and locked him in his trunk. They used his cab to transport drugs through the night. As he lay in the dark, Arturo made a promise to God in exchange for survival. Thinking of his relatives who had converted to evangelical Protestantism and "always carried their Bibles with them," he told God that he would convert. He also swore to "be a better husband and father" if he lived. At dawn, the carjackers opened the trunk, and one prepared to shoot Arturo in the head. He pulled the trigger, but the gun jammed. The men got scared and ran off, leaving him alive. Arturo believed this was divine intervention.

Five years later, I sat with Arturo and his wife, Ade, around a desk in a medical examination cubicle. We were in the Cuernavaca office of the Human Papillomavirus in Men (HIM) study, a multinational observational research project funded by the National Institutes of Health that tracks the occurrence of that sexually transmitted virus in male research subjects over time. Ade was trim, with short, stylish gray hair and a French manicure. Arturo was also graying, but stockier, dressed smartly in a polo shirt and crisp khakis. The talkative couple were quick to laugh and complement each other and eager to discuss the intimate and sometimes painful experiences they had lived through. Arturo's brush with death was one of the worst; Ade recalled waiting as he failed to come home, hopefully imagining nonlethal reasons such as car trouble but fearing the worst amid the rash of violent crime. Yet they also said the experience led to positive changes for Arturo as a man and for them both as a couple. Arturo kept his promises to God, converting and striving to keep up with the emerging local ideal of emotionally open masculinity by being a more dedicated, caring and present spouse and parent.

His enrollment in the HIM study was a part of that transformation. Ade had heard about the HIM study in her work as a nurse at the Instituto Mexicano del Seguro Social (IMSS), the federal health agency that administered the study in Mexico. She suggested that he join, since it seemed in keeping with his new emphasis on caring for his family and helping others. They believed that Arturo's getting tested for the often-asymptomatic human papillomavirus (HPV) would protect both his and Ade's health, as well as that of other people. Ade said, "You're supporting an investigation, right? That can help to prevent [bad] experiences for people down the line." Arturo added that the international study could have "a benefit for the whole world." It could also model a way to be manly by helping others in ways that countered his attackers' violent and careless masculinity. The couple saw Arturo's participation in medical research as a way to care for themselves, help others, and help him to be the new kind of man he wanted to be.

In this book I follow middle-class, heterosexual couples such as Ade and Arturo through four years of men's participation in the Cuernavaca HIM study. Longitudinal, observational medical research such as the HIM study does not test clinical interventions. Instead, it uses repeated clinical testing to assess change over time in participants' bodies. This kind of medical research takes up only a small part of a participant's daily life. Yet it can be consequential. For example, when a man unexpectedly tests positive for an asymptomatic HPV infection, it can cause marital problems and lead to fear about his partners' vulnerability to HPV-related cervical cancer. However, as for Arturo, research participation can also help a man live out his goal of helping others and enable him to care for his and his spouse's sexual health.

Medical research designers and regulators generally understand participation as an individual experience with largely biological consequences. Participants' bodies are the primary objects of medical study. Participants' contexts—such as Arturo's close-knit marriage and traumatic encounter with rising narcoviolence—are seen as biologically relevant only in terms of how they influence participants' health and adherence to study protocols. Yet a rich body of social-science work shows that context matters deeply for participants' research experiences, which can be profoundly social, as well as physical. This work also critiques the idea that participants are passive "human subjects" of research. Research that focuses especially on impoverished and marginalized people's immersion in the globalized world of clinical trials has demonstrated how people often actively seek inclusion in studies and use research experiences to pursue broader life goals.

Those insights inspired my research into the ways that middle-class, unpaid participants might incorporate longitudinal observational research into their broader life projects. What it means economically and structurally to be "middle class" varies widely. Yet the term identifies a shared subject position from which people who understand themselves as precariously economically mobile and capable of creating change have driven the spread of self-consciously modern ideals and practices, adopting and promoting new forms of marriage, worship, and health behavior (cf. Freeman 2014). While HIM participants and their partners had varying levels of economic stability, they shared an understanding of themselves as secure enough to work toward societal change yet poor enough to be free of the corrupt self-absorption they attributed to Mexico's elite. Here, I investigate how people sought to meet both class-based economic needs and social goals in part through participation in medical research.

I analyze how people's cultural ideologies regarding health—including gender, race, and the fundamental nature of personhood—not only influenced their own experiences of medical research, but actually enabled them to incorporate research participation into wide-ranging social and biological goals at the levels of the couple, the family, and the Mexican populace. Amid violent instability and government inaction, middle-class HIM study participants sought venues for doing good that came to include medical research enrollment. I found that couples hoped to change their own and others' lives for the better through men's unpaid participation in HPV research. This hope depended on a fundamental rejection of the idea that medical research was an individual pursuit. I contend that this rejection reflected a local cultural ideology of personhood that cast Mexicans as members of a racially interrelated social and biological whole rather than as members of a society composed of a collection of individuals. They saw themselves as components of what I call a "collective biology"—an interconnected biosocial group whose behavior and biology could be altered via the actions of constituent parts of the larger whole.

I argue that HIM participants' and their partners' understandings of their bodies and society as collective rather than individual fundamentally influenced their study experiences. This ideology enabled them to incorporate research participation into broader efforts to improve their own and others' lives. They did not share the HIM study's emphasis on men's individual bodies as the key site of change to be monitored. Instead, they understood social bodies, at the levels of the couple, the family, the church, and the Mexican nation, as both metaphorical and literal entities that they could positively influence through men's participation in medical research. As middle-class research volunteers in a society intent on modernization but suffering from violent crisis, these couples incorporated men's HIM experiences into ongoing attempts to be "good" people and couples. They hoped to care for their families by raising children to emulate desirable gender and health behavior and to advance Mexican society by modeling modernity despite the chaos of narcoviolence and government unreliability.

Further, because they saw themselves as parts of these larger biosocial wholes, they expected their modern comportment and health behavior to actually improve the health of these collective bodies from within. This belief that men's HPV testing could have such far-reaching consequences depended on a collectivist understanding of human biology, which emphasized the effects that individuals' changes might have for group health and well-being. While the often highly educated study participants generally understood how human papillomavirus functioned in men's individual bodies, they cared more about its effects on what they saw as the collective biologies of the couple, the family, and a Mexican national body that they believed to be physically interrelated through a shared racial heritage.

This analysis also serves to develop the concept of collective biologies itself. It extends the anthropologist Margaret Lock's foundational concept of "local biologies": the idea that human biology is not the universal assumed in biomedicine but, instead, context-specific and arising from "ongoing dialectic[s] between biology and culture in which both are contingent" (Lock 1993: xxi; Lock and Kaufert 2001). While careless applications of this concept risk reproducing biologically essentialist and scientifically invalid racial or class typologies (Meloni 2014; Niewöhner and Lock 2018; Yates-

Doerr 2017), applying it with appropriate nuance enables us to understand how the material and social aspects of varying histories and contexts differently shapes the development of human bodies (Brotherton and Nguyen 2013; Lock and Nguyen 2018)—including their assessment via medical screening (Burke 2014).

Here I extend this approach to examine a cultural factor that influenced the health behavior—and, thus, ultimately the local biologies—of medical research participants in Mexico. That factor is the idea that the "social body," a productive metaphor long used to understand societies (e.g., Scheper-Hughes and Lock 1987; Wilkis 2015), might not always be just metaphorical. In some cases social bodies are composed of literally biologically interrelated entities. I identify such units as collective biologies and provide a model for using that concept to investigate how people incorporate nonindividual understandings of biology into their health behavior and life choices. This approach extends a line of ethnographic work within the rubric of feminist new materialisms, which analyzes how people's lived experiences of emergent medical technologies serve as context-contingent sites for the coproduction of specific forms of biology and social life (Roberts 2016).

Thus, this book also extends the scope of social-science research on the experience of medical research participation. Studies of this arena have focused productively on the experiences of participants motivated by structural and social marginalization to enroll in shorter-term, medically invasive clinical trials (see, e.g., Fisher 2020). Here I investigate middle-class couples' simultaneously physical and social hopes for participation in long-term, longitudinal observational medical research that monitors rather than alters people's bodies. Most HIM participants were partnered with women, and couples often participated in joint decision making about enrollment. For example, many talked together with staff to understand the meaning of men's test results for both partners. To reflect this reality, and to resist beginning from the assumption that medical research participation was a fundamentally individual act, I took couples rather than individuals as my primary unit of analysis.

Love and marriage are key life arenas for living out both old and new social ideals and reproducing them through child rearing (Ahearn 2001; Hirsch et al. 2009; Hunter 2010; Povinelli 2006). Focusing on couples thus allowed me to investigate how people collaborated to incorporate men's research participation into shared daily life projects. This focus enabled analysis of the ways that people's efforts to live out local ideals of gender and race, which include assumptions that people are heterosexual and will reproduce, influenced their experiences of and belief in the transformative possibilities of sexual health research. I found that romantic partnerships represented the innermost circle in the series of biosocial bodies that couples believed men's medical research participation could influence. In this book, I take these partnerships as my starting point for investigating the ways that people sought to incorporate study participation into collective biologies at the levels of the couple, the family, the church, and the nation.

My analysis shows that despite medical studies' framing as individual and exploratory, participants can understand them as treatment for simultaneously biological and social ills on the level of the social as well as the individual body. These findings extend the social-science insight that the "human subjects" who participate in medical research can, in fact, be very active agents and that the relationships in which they are enmeshed—with people, ideas, and economic and cultural context—fundamentally shape how they experience and make social use of research participation. Further, they make the new contribution of revealing how culturally specific ideas about the nature of these relationships—in the Mexican case, as simultaneously biological and social—influence people's hopes for, behavior within, and understandings of medical research participation. They also broaden the scope of our understandings of the consequences and possibilities for medical research and of the global landscape that has made it increasingly common. Most social-science work on this topic has investigated the experiences of poor and marginalized research participants. Here I examine how middle-class, heterosexual Mexicans who see themselves as the backbone of their society look to health research to treat social and biological ills simultaneously.

Given the central role that debates about good masculinities and femininities play in current Mexican discussions of modernity and race, my analysis expands our current understanding of research participation by focusing on its gendered and racialized aspects. I analyze the ways that middle-class participants hoped their self-consciously modern performances of health care, progressive masculinity, and modern marriage would enhance the well-being of broader biosocial wholes at multiple levels, from the couple to the Mexican social body. I show that they hoped to create change in two main ways. They sought to model ideally modern Mexicanness that would encourage others in the populace to engage in health-enhancing behavior. They also cared for their own physical health in ways they hoped would directly improve the health of the loved ones they slept with and cared for. These findings further reveal how in a context of national upheaval, medical research participation became a way that people sought to be good citizens and lead their nation forward, in spite of government failings.

These insights can help us improve medical research design, analysis, and oversight. For instance, they demonstrate that participants' cultural ideas about biology and health directly influence both their desire to enroll in medical research and the potentially widespread biosocial consequences of that enrollment. These findings are key for research recruitment and ethics oversight. In addition, they can also help us think beyond business as usual in medical research. The design and assessment of medical research and public health projects would look different if individuals were understood as interrelated parts of a collective biology. In settings where people hold this cultural ideology, assessing exactly how they hope their own health behavior will treat others' ills can provide health workers with a guide for creating such change. Health researchers and public health workers can use participants' own ideas about how one's actions influence the biosocial whole as a model for both assessing and creating societal-level effects of individual health practice.

Medical Research as Relational Experience

Medical research looks very different depending on the worldview of the person studying it. Medical research designers and regulators worldwide follow guidelines developed out of the 1978 U.S. Belmont Report as they engage with research participants. The Belmont Report was a response to prior abuses, such as the Tuskegee syphilis study and Nazi experimentation, intended to identify ways to protect the "human subjects" of medical research. As such, the report and the concept of participants as "subjects" frame researchers as actively protecting or harming people, who more passively respond to research experiences. The report's findings also reflect specifically Anglo-American cultural ideas about the nature of personhood that have spread around the world along with the globalization of medical research (Petryna 2009; Stark 2011). The report understands "human subjects" as "autonomous agents," reflecting American ideals of independence and individuality by defining respect for people's autonomy as the ability to freely make decisions on their own (Sims 2010). A key aim of regulation in this model is to avoid the "therapeutic misconception," in which people confuse the aims of medical research with the aims of clinical care and believe that studies are designed to treat them rather than generate knowledge (Dresser 2002). From this perspective, the only safe and legitimate reason for participating in research is the altruistic desire to help the unspecified others who might benefit from scientific advances, rather than to directly benefit oneself or one's loved ones (Montoya 2011).

However, social-science researchers who investigate how people's diverse contexts influence their research experiences have shown that this individualistic and biologically focused view is often inaccurate. For example, it fails to account for the fact that many aspects of identity that participants see as central to their experience of research—such as gender and one's place within a family—are developed through interactions with others (Sariola and Simpson 2011). An individualistic focus obscures how participants' interpersonal relationships mediate clinical outcomes—for instance, by influencing how participants comply with study protocols (Scott et al. 2011). It also takes for granted the American cultural notion of autonomy as individuality, which does not apply in societies where people value collaborative decision making with others. For instance, deciding jointly that Arturo would participate in the HIM study was central for his and Ade's experience, providing a way for her to share in and support his lifestyle change. While critical feminist bioethicists have long called for attention to the relationality inherent in participants' decision making officially idealized as "autonomous" (Meynell and Borgerson 2020; Sherwin 1998: 19), consent processes that attend to such lived relationality remain experimental and marginal to institutional bioethics oversight of medical research (cf. Ramabu 2019).

Nevertheless, research reveals that, in contrast to the assumption of "human subjects'" experiences as individual and impersonal, people worldwide often use participation in clinical trials to pursue wide-ranging social ends (Fisher 2013). For instance, participation can be a way to assert desired attributes such as respectability, virtue, selflessness, or expertise to others (Black 2019; Dixon and Tameris 2018; Stadler et al. 2018). This aim can be woven into the broader moral projects of daily life beyond the clinic, such as quitting stigmatized behavior such as smoking (Wolters et al. 2014). Thus, people can assert specific identities through participation in medical research. This is similarly true for participation in other forms of health surveillance, such as screening programs (Armstrong 2005, 2019).

People may also forge new kinds of relationships through research participation that reflect and respond to the forms of inequality that shape clinical trial worlds (Fisher 2020). Forming and maintaining bonds of trust between researchers and participants is necessary for the research process (Compaoré et al. 2018; Thabethe et al. 2018). Yet these relationships can range much more widely, from participants' reconceptualizations of researchers as caregivers (Leach and Fairhead 2011; Reynolds et al. 2013) to the creation of new study-based communities and forms of kinship (Geissler et al. 2008) that can persist long after experiments end (Nguyen 2015). Medical research participation can be an active site for the creation of new social forms and cultural meanings, such as affiliation with political subcultures (Abadie 2010) or new forms of valuation (Swallow et al. 2020). It can serve to create and relate people to life-shaping identity categories such as racial or ethnic labels (Epstein 2008a, 2008b; Valdez 2019). Participation can also be a site for advocating for attention to marginalized groups' concerns and for staking broader rights claims (Epstein 1996).

The anthropologist Susan Reynolds Whyte (2011: 49) thus argues that, to fully understand this aspect of human experience, "We should be asking how relationships are developed, expressed and mediated in medical research." This makes sense, given the findings discussed above and the fact that, despite the American cultural fixation on individuality, people's daily life experiences of making ethical choices include consideration of how their actions will affect others' interrelated social and physical futures (Al-Mohammad 2010; Csordas 2008; Weiss 1999). Indeed, providing biological or experiential data for medical research can be part of a broader, daily life process of making meaning and seeking to do right within one's interpersonal relationships (Sheikh and Jensen 2019).

Since sexual reproduction so obviously requires human interaction, clinical trials of contraception highlight how people's research experiences actually depend on their relationships. While the effects of medical research participation on gender are rarely studied, two scholars have shown that clinical trials can be sites in which people collaborate with romantic partners, and even researchers, to construct and perform ideals of gender and love. Nelly Oudshoorn's (2003) research on studies of oral contraceptives for men revealed that participants, their female partners, and study researchers understood the project as affecting the couple as a whole, given the risk of pregnancy. Further, female partners and researchers collaborated to frame male pill testers as performers of simultaneously adventuresome and progressive masculinities. Similarly, Catherine Montgomery's (2012) analysis of women's experiences in a microbicide trial showed that, while study designers imagined subjects gaining autonomy thorough confidential contraceptive use, participants themselves worked with their partners to use the technology to pursue shared sexual benefits and to strengthen their romantic relationships. These examples highlight that relationships with other people (such as spouses) and with elements of broader context (such as gender ideals) fundamentally influence participants' actions and experiences of research. They further show that participants might understand medical research as affecting their embodied relationships rather than just their individual biologies.

Participants' relationships to the structural aspects of their context—the economic and political setting that determines the conditions of their daily lives—also fundamentally shape their experiences of medical research. Qualitative research shows that participants might see their relationships with study staff as economic exchange or labor, as they trade bodily substances for care or compensation (Alenichev and Nguyen 2019; Cooper and Waldby 2014; Fairhead et al. 2006; Nguyen 2015). This is quite different from the regulatory ideal of participating for altruism rather than personal gain. Yet it reflects the fact that making decisions without constraint is a privilege that few people have in an unequal world. Economic need and the widespread harms faced by members of marginalized groups influence people's decisions to participate in medical research (Gaut 1995; Montoya 2011; Towghi and Vora 2014). For instance, in contexts where international nongovernmental organizations are key sources of employment, research participation can thus be an entrepreneurial act in which people balance fears of exploitation with hopes that it will offer new economic opportunities with trial sponsors (Bruun 2016). Further, when people lack money and access to care the so-called therapeutic misconception that medical research delivers health care might not be incorrect after all. While medical research is not intended to improve participants' health, it sometimes offers the only health screening or care people can get (Fisher 2008; Molyneux et al. 2005; Montoya 2011; Reynolds et al. 2013; Waldby 2012).

This phenomenon is especially powerful as medical clinical trials increasingly enroll poor and marginalized populations worldwide. Members of such groups often rely on participation for income or basic health care (Elliott and Abadie 2008; Farmer 2002; Fisher 2008, 2013; Geissler 2013; Kamat 2014; Nguyen 2009; Petryna 2009). This reality is generally unacknowledged by local Institutional Review Boards that follow the American focus on individuals abstracted from context (Simpson et al. 2015), even if participants and local research workers are quite aware of it (Rayzberg 2019). Structural context matters for even economically stable participants' experiences, as with Ade and Arturo's experience of violent insecurity that made HIM participation attractive. It also shapes study staff members' motivations as workers, as they might hope to aid their communities by securing international support for local industry and infrastructure (Genus 2018). In light of these relationships, some scholars call for understanding research projects and the communities that host them as intertwined systems rather than separate entities (Wyss-van den Berg et al. 2020).

These dynamics of interdependence occur in other situations in which entities from the global North seek data from groups that lack resources. Lauren Carruth (2018) demonstrates this in the case of data collection by international humanitarian organizations in the Somali region of Ethiopia. There, potential beneficiaries of aid and local data collectors develop evolving strategies for seeking support from humanitarian "audit culture" itself, which include attendant changes in their forms of interaction and presentations of self. These power-laden relationships among aid organizations, local workers, and research participants/potential beneficiaries fundamentally shape the design and interpretation of health research studies, as well (Biruk 2011, 2018).

By investigating the ways that HIM participants and their partners' relationships to people and their contexts influenced their medical research experiences, I follow Sassy Molyneux and P. Wenzel Geissler's call to understand research participants' experiences holistically rather than individualistically by examining them at different "levels of scale" (Molyneux and Geissler 2008: 687). These levels span the interpersonal and the societal, in an approach that, Geissler (2011: 6) writes, "destabilizes taken-for-granted boundaries" in the study of medical research participation by refocusing the object of inquiry beyond the individual participants' biologies and experiences. This approach builds on the fundamental medical anthropological insight that health experiences cannot be fully understood without analysis of how they affect a person's physically felt body; social relationships; *and* interactions with laws, policies, and other aspects of social structure (Scheper-Hughes and Lock 1987). In the case of medical research, attending to multiple levels of scale enables study of how participants' research experiences fit into the rich webs of physical and social interactions with people, cultural ideologies, and structural contexts that make up their lives.

In this book, I investigate the ways that HIM participation matters for people's embodied relationships at the levels of scale that they cared about most. My analysis traces how HIM participants and their partners made men's HPV testing matter at the levels of the couple, the family and church, and the Mexican nation. Analyzing the HIM study experience at multiple levels of scale enables me to faithfully capture couples' experiences of participation as nonindividual and as both socially and physically consequential for the collective biologies to which they belonged. My goal is to provide a holistic rather than individualistic view of the complex reasons that men participated in the HIM study, and of the wide range of collective biosocial benefits they and their partners sought, on the various levels of scale that came to matter in this Mexican context. I hope that this analysis will provide a model for understanding the concrete consequences of medical research participation for collective rather than individual bodies, which medical research designers and regulators can use to broaden their ideas of harms and benefits from the individual "human subject" to the participant's physically and socially interconnected world.

The Setting

MESTIZAJE AND IDEAS OF THE MEXICAN SOCIAL BODY

People's hopes that their individual participation in the HIM study would have widespread benefits draw implicitly on an ideology of collective "Mexicanness" embodied in the concept of *mestizaje* (mixing). In Mexico, it is commonly believed that Spanish conquest of Indigenous peoples began a process of racial mixing that would beget a racially and culturally unique *mestizo* (mixed) population. Governments since conquest have promoted engagement in the behavior and body practices desired by elites as ways for people to shed Indianness and assimilate into more privileged racial categories aligned with whiteness and Europeanness (Alonso 2004; Knight 1990). Postrevolutionary federal programs and public intellectuals then fused ideologies of mixing with nationalism to promote biological and cultural homogenization into an idealized mestizo populace imagined to be ideally suited for citizenship. These efforts popularized the idea that the Mexican social body is interrelated in two intertwined ways: through a shared racial heritage of ethnic mixture, and through a common societal aim of evolving toward the ideal behavioral expression of that mestizo identity.

This ideology of race conflicts with the anthropological view that the concept of race is not scientifically valid. Anthropologists argue that there are no essentially biologically different human groups, and the biological variation among people assigned any racial category is just as great as the variation between people assigned to different categories (Fuentes et al. 2019). Instead, we argue that race is a cultural ideology with immense power to affect people's lives and, in turn, their bodies. It is from this perspective that I analyze the ideology of Mexican mestizaje as an element of cultural context that shapes HIM participants' experiences.

Currently dominant ideas about race in Mexico continue to reflect revolution-era takes on this notion of mestizaje. The Mexican Revolution (ca. 1910–20) entailed complex interactions among varied political factions representing diverse groups and forged new national political and cultural ideologies. It ushered in a new constitution in 1917, marking an era in which the goal of government was reconceptualized as serving the needs of a national population imagined as a cohesive whole. Politicians and public intellectuals promoted of a specific kind of Mexican mestizaje as part of efforts to create a homogeneous, governable, and modern national populace in this new political landscape (Alonso 2004; Manrique 2017).

José Vasconcelos, minister of education in the early 1920s, most clearly articulated this vision in his notion of Mexicans as *la raza cósmica*. He asserted that Indigenous and European populations present in Mexico would mix over time into a "cosmic race" ideally suited for modernity (Vasconcelos [1925] 1997). He and his contemporaries promoted this ideology widely. For example, Vasconcelos supported the famous Mexican muralist movement comprising painters such as Diego Rivera, which romanticized indigeneity but framed it not as an end goal but as a contributor toward a mestizo future (Manrique 2016). This ideology also extended and influenced Mexican eugenicists' efforts to frame hybridity, rather than "purity," as the racial trait that would produce more biologically and socially fit populations (Stepan 1991). The idea that a cohesive Mexican social body was coming into physical and social existence, and that it could be strengthened and advanced by disciplining Indian bodies and behavior into whiter, mestizo-identified comportment, has been represented in literature and promoted in schools for over a century (Janzen 2015; Sierra [1900] 1969; Vaughan 1997; Vaughan and Lewis 2006; Walsh 2004).

This idea that racial mixture combined with ideal behavior could create a better population has animated national public health projects from the revolution through today. Government health programs have framed health practices as ways to embody modern mestizaje, behaviorally and— through the effects of that behavior on the body—biologically. These efforts have also emphasized the performance of ideal gender norms as key to health, modernity, and the creation of new generations who would embody these traits (González-Santos 2020). For example, twentieth-century health campaigns sought to teach parents to rear children who would form the new, ideal population (Stern 2003). Framing families as microcosms of both nation and "race" has been a common way to align embodied practices of gender with emerging societal-level goals, while often perpetuating foundational inequalities (see, e.g., Pirinjian 2019; Stoler 1989). Mexican visions of the "revolutionary family" tasked women, as mothers, with physically and morally nurturing future citizens by instilling hygienic behavior in children (Stern 1999) and men, as fathers, with transmitting state goals to their families while eliminating unhealthy and unproductive behavior coded as Indigenous, such as binge drinking (Bliss 1999; Joseph et al. 2001). Physicians even predicted that mestiza women's pelvises would reach an ideal midpoint between too-narrow European and too-wide Indigenous structures, reflecting stereotypes about each group's femininity and the kind of womanhood that would enable national progress (Cházaro 2005). These racial ideologies and gendered expectations of women's responsibility for the healthy reproduction of the nation have become intrinsic to the Mexican state and its systems (Sue 2013). They now underlie representations of the Mexican population, from federal genomic health research (Saldaña-Tejeda 2018a) to the national forensic database (Nieves Delgado 2020) and pornography (Mezo Gonzalez 2018).

They also fuel persistent, racialized inequalities. Such ideologies of mixing have created and reinforced the racial categories understood as the base components of mixture (Wade 2004). For example, the category of "Indian" resulted from the homogenization of diverse pre-Columbian societies into one subjugated group amid conquest. It is an inherent driver of racialized inequality and marginalization. Given this context, the varied ideologies of mestizaje that emerged throughout post-conquest Latin America have always framed "Indian" and "European" (and, in some cases, "African") as discrete racial groups that all mix together but are unequally valued in a process of homogenization hoped to entail physical and behavioral whitening (Chaves and Zambrano 2006; Stepan 1991; Wade 2004).

This is true even for utopian visions of mestizaje. Vasconcelos ([1925] 1997) wrote about racial mixing as a move toward a fully intermixed, ideal, and thus equal population. Yet efforts to promote Mexican mestizaje have always centered a Europeanized or whitened mestizo as the emblem of modernity and, in the process, have both perpetuated and concealed systemic, racialized inequalities (Manrique 2016). This powerful ideology of mestizaje is dominant enough to write out the presence of populations who identify with heritage other than the Indigenous and European components thought to contribute to la raza cósmica. For instance, government genetics programs currently define the "Mexican population" as mestizo (López-Beltrán and Deister 2013). The category of Afro-Mexican was added to national government population surveys only in 2015, following activists' efforts to challenge dominant narratives about the nation's racial composition (Love 2015; Vaughn 2013).

Thus, I interpret urban, non-Indigenous research participants' frequent use of the term "Mexican" to discuss their own identities and natures as indexing this culturally ubiquitous understanding of "Mexican" as mestizo/a. When I discuss mestizaje as an implicit conceptual underpinning for participants' explicit narratives of their medical research experiences, I am also acknowledging their favored position within a national system of racial hierarchy that oppresses Indigenous people and others who do not culturally or phenotypically match elite visions of mestizo Mexicanness. Like whiteness in the United States, claiming the identity of "Mexican" provides social privilege, as this is understood to be the default, "normal," and ideal category of personhood by those with the most social power (Moreno Figueroa 2010).

Yet unlike North American notions of whiteness, the category of mestizo refers to an always ongoing process rather than a static, essential trait or group. First, the notion of racial mixing toward perfection imagines a future in which race will cease to exist, as everyone is mestizo. So while there are still "Indians," the process of mestizaje is incomplete. Importantly, it always will be, since, as mentioned earlier, ideologies of mestizaje also continually reproduce the racial categories understood to be the components of mixture (Wade 2004). Second, race in this framework is both biological—an essence transmitted through ancestry—and, even more important, behavioral. As I show, HIM participants' narratives about their responsibility to a social body reflect how mestizaje works as an aspirational and ongoing body project.

Thus, having lighter skin is just one way to access privilege. People can also claim mestizo status by acting in ways classed as modern (implicitly, oriented toward Europeanness or whiteness) versus "traditional" (explicitly, Indian) (Perez Lopez 2017). While Latin American countries have different national racial ideologies, throughout the region whitening and belonging in privileged racial categories is attainable through behavior (de la Cadena 2008), including health behavior (cf. Roberts 2006). Interventions such as the Mexican public health and education campaigns discussed earlier have long fostered the belief that individuals' actions can define them as either "decent people" or not; decent meaning mestizo rather than Indian, middle versus lower class, and respectable versus disreputable (Hind 2017). So mestizaje is something one does, by embracing current cultural ideals of modernity and rejecting stigmatized behavior associated with indigeneity. Further, it is something one does in the name of the collective social body. The idea that anyone in Mexico can join the racial category of mestizo through "modern" behavior, and should do so to advance the nation, enables discrimination against Indigenous-identified and darker-skinned people to be dismissed not as racism, but as the consequence of those people's own failure to assimilate (Moreno Figueroa and Saldívar Tanaka 2015; Saldívar 2014).

For example, implicitly mestizo-identified health workers often critique patients' behavior and self-presentation they see as antimodern, unhygienic, or backwardly Indigenous (Gutiérrez Chong 2017; Smith-Oka 2012). As with the broader discourse of mestizaje that reifies the racial categories it purports to supersede, medical education in Mexico fuses stated ideals of providing care for the nation with systems that reinforce providers' privileged class and racial status relative to the public service users who provide raw material for their training (Smith-Oka and Marshalla 2019). Thus, in Cuernavaca, government health workers often place the blame for poor and less-educated people's failure to perform preventative health care on an implicitly Indian or low-class "culture of ignorance" that they, as more educated citizens, have the duty to combat (Schneider 2010). Health campaigns continue to target antimodern behavior framed as the product of Indigenous or lower-class cultures while obscuring state failures to reduce the poverty and inequality that most significantly determine health opportunities (Soto Laveaga 2007).

In keeping with that emphasis on personal behavior as the key to national modernization, middle-class mestizos often cast their own sociomedical practices as ways to promote progress in the social body and offset the negative contributions of Indigenous or low-income others. For instance, Lara Braff (2013) found that non-Indigenous fertility clinic patients in Mexico City engaged in "reproductive othering." They criticized rural, Indigenous, and poor women for contributing to overpopulation and transmitting backward cultural views. In contrast, they and their physicians justified their own efforts to reproduce by framing themselves as prepared, modern, and implicitly whiter than those imagined others. Their use of medicine as an arena for such assertions makes particular sense since Mexican medical systems— especially specialties related to reproductive health and pediatrics—were developed to deliberately improve and modernize the national populace (González-Santos 2020).

This use of assisted reproduction to assert elite status and imbue a next generation with it demonstrates the processuality inherent in Mexican mestizaje. As the presumptive progeny of Indigenous and European ancestors, members of this group can act in ways that are more closely aligned with the imagined characteristics of either racial pole, facilitating or thwarting the embodied and cultural whitening over time in the Mexican social body. Thus, while projects promoting gender and health modernities to facilitate governance have been common worldwide (see, e.g., Adams and Pigg 2005; Briggs 2002; Hunt 1999), in Mexico they have reflected and reified the ideal of a population moving toward increasing biological and cultural homogeneity. Practices of ideal gender and health behavior are thus ways of aligning more and more with modernity over time in the service of developing a national, mestizo collective.

This racial ideology also profoundly influenced HIM participants' experiences. Their hopes that men's research participation could benefit broader biosocial bodies drew on the idea that Mexicans as mestizos share a unique biological and cultural essence that, if lived out well, could advance the Mexican race and nation. It is important to note that participants did not speak of themselves as mestizo, as is typical of members of a dominant and culturally unmarked racial category. Instead, they frequently and self-consciously referred to themselves as "Mexican." Given the pervasiveness and longevity of the ideology of mestizaje, I interpret self-identification as Mexican during discussions of population modernity or ideal behavior as drawing implicitly on the beliefs discussed earlier. This is not to say that all participants supported such a vision of Mexicanness, could articulate histories of its construction or promotion, or thought consciously about it. Instead, I argue that the common pattern of participants' referring to themselves and others as "Mexican" to explain their characters, bodies, and behavior drew meaning from this shared cultural history regarding the nature of "Mexicanness" as mestizaje, albeit in implicit and varied ways. They used the term especially to reference the ambivalence inherent to concepts of Mexicanness: that it entailed both innate urges toward backward behavior and the behavioral possibility of advancing beyond it.

This was evident in Arturo and Ade's understandings of what Arturo's study participation could achieve. The couple felt that the study was beneficial to them specifically "as Mexicans." Both saw preventative health care as valuable but said that they suffered from what they saw as an innate cultural predisposition to avoid it. Discussing how their efforts to eat healthily were hampered by Arturo's periods of unemployment, and the cheapness and temptation of tortillas and rice, Ade she said that failing to care for one's health was "the idiosyncrasy of this country." She explained, "We're

lazy, right? As Mexicans, we're more about correcting than preventing. . . .
We're not very farsighted." They discussed HIM participation as a way to
work against this instinct.

I argue that the rhetorical choice to frame these problems as issues inherent to Mexicans draws clearly, if implicitly, on the ideology of mestizaje
discussed earlier. Mestizaje is never a completed project. It must be accomplished by ongoing rejection of the backward, implicitly Indigenous tendencies within one's mixed constitution. Such rejection requires behavioral
alignment with an implicitly whiter, modern future. Further, it is a set of
individual choices culturally framed as reflecting and affecting the evolution
of the Mexican populace.

For Ade, to be Mexican is thus to be innately pulled in both progressive
and regressive directions. Her ongoing efforts to act in modern ways—for
example, by engaging in preventative health care—demonstrate privileged
racial status on the individual level and hold the promise of moving the populace as a whole forward on the imagined continuum toward realizing the
potential of la raza cósmica. This ideology was typical of HIM participants
who saw themselves as predisposed to regressive behaviors because of their
Mexicanness, as well as made vulnerable by the Mexican nation's economic
failings, but also understood actions such as research participation as a way
to begin with themselves to create change in the social body and help their
nation advance. Throughout this book, I investigate the ways such hopes
motivated medical research participation.

Gender in the Social Body

As demonstrated by the foci of national public health projects, gender norms
have been closely linked with cultural visions of ideal Mexicanness. While
women have been tasked with demonstrating ideal mestiza femininity to
raise modern and healthy families, men have been simultaneously feared
to reflect the worst of Mexicanness and exhorted to embody its best. The
macho form of masculinity stereotypically identified with Mexican men developed out of revolutionary-era political and media rhetoric linking the
essence of the new Mexican nation to a tough and respectable but violent
form of masculinity (Alonso 1995). The notion that Mexican men share an
innate *machismo* has become culturally ingrained since the 1950s and persists,
despite critiques that themselves have been widespread since the 1990s (Gutmann 1996). With the internal complexity and conflict that characterizes
most cultural ideologies, this trait is attributed simultaneously to the notion

that mestizo men's conquistador ancestry made them innately predisposed to womanizing, violence, and emotional withdrawal and that their Indigenous ancestry inclines them to forms of social backwardness, including in their styles of masculinity (Melhuus 1996; Paz [1961] 1985).

Thus, machismo is a cultural idea rather than an accurate descriptor of most men's identity. Nevertheless, it remains a central way that Mexicans understand masculinities (Domínguez-Ruvalcaba 2007; McKee Irwin 2003). Machismo has long and fiercely been critiqued as a barrier to national advancement and gender equity (Amuchástegui Herrera and Szasz 2007; Gutmann 1996; Ramirez 2009). Today, the term "machismo" is seen as negative even by male gang members who value violent toughness alongside specific forms of protectiveness and care (Sverdlin 2017). Even as male violence is increasing in a context of economic inequality and insecurity that makes forms of care such as breadwinning increasingly difficult to perform (Gamlin and Hawkes 2017), men and boys from varied walks of life critique what is now seen as a problematically "traditional" form of manhood (Singleton et al. 2018). These contradictions reflect simultaneous challenges to and maintenance of Mexican gender stereotypes (Galeana and Vargas Becerra 2015) within a context that the sociologist Gloria González-López (2015: 20) calls "a changing and unpredictable patriarchal collage."

Yet these common critiques of machismo still often frame it as a natural attribute of Mexican men. In contexts from antiviolence classes to medical care, people call for men to struggle against their presumptively innate tendencies toward violence and womanizing (Amuchástegui Herrera 2008; Wentzell 2013). This idea of an inherently problematic Mexican masculinity is also continuously revitalized by discourses about Mexican womanhood. Women's claims to rights often invoke rather than disrupt ideals of femininity forged during the Mexican Revolution, which fuse even earlier emphases on domesticity with valorization of toughness and resilience. Women's strength and participation in the public sphere are made palatable via emphases on mothering, caring for one's family, fidelity, and the ability to *aguantar* (suffer through) adversity, including that dealt by macho men (Haney 2012; Melero 2015; Melhuus 1996). Thus, even as people decry machismo, they keep the concept alive by framing their own behavior and experience in relationship to it (Gutmann 1996; Ramirez 2009).

Alongside this enduring assumption about Mexican men's problematic nature, new ideals of marriage and masculinity have emerged. In Cuernavaca, gender roles and relationships have become more egalitarian over the past several decades (LeVine 1993). Critiques of machismo and calls for "modern" gender norms are now common. They include calls for the increasingly globally popular experience of "companionate marriage." This is a self-consciously modern form of marriage centered on love, intimacy, and mutual pleasure rather than economic production or biological reproduction (Hirsch 2003; Padilla et al. 2007; Wardlow and Hirsch 2006). While strong and lasting extended family ties have long been a Mexican cultural ideal, people now often emphasize love and the ability to develop personally within a supportive nuclear family structure as key to the maintenance of such bonds (Nehring 2011). Yet it is important to note that companionate forms of marriage and masculinity reconfigure, but do not erase, gendered forms of hierarchy and power (Shakuto 2019). While for some companionate marriage represents a modernization of gender roles in comparison with a "traditional" past, and may also represent modernity in that same-sex marriage is now legally recognized throughout Mexico, it is also a subject of activist critique as an institution that upholds antiquated forms of gender, sexual, and social organization and the economic arrangements on which they rest (cf. Russo Garrido 2020).

The currently dominant ideal of companionate marriage in Mexico also reflects preexisting racial hierarchies. Specific ideologies of marriage have long been associated with modernity and mestizaje, but their content has changed over time. At one time, having separate spheres for women and men defined families as mestizo rather than Indigenous (Browner 1989). Now, companionate marriage exemplifies visions of modernity associated with *blanqueamiento* (whitening), which reject machismo, separate spheres, and emphasis on reproduction in favor of a focus on couple's intimacy (Ramirez and Everett 2018).

In practice, people today widely desire what researchers call companionate marriage, but they understand it diversely. Such notions of good marriage vary from explicitly feminist egalitarianism to coupling respect for women with the maintenance of patriarchy. Yet whatever gender expectations people have for their own marriages, they usually define them in contrast to "traditional" forms of marriage and masculinity, which they frame as barriers to both national modernization and personal fulfillment (see, e.g., Wentzell 2013).

While emphasis on successful provision has remained central to understandings of positive manliness in Mexico and elsewhere (cf. Smith 2017), ideals of men's responsibility have broadened to incorporate provision of care and intimacy, including care for one's self through health behavior

(Amuchástegui Herrera and Szasz 2007; de Keijzer 2016; Gutmann 2007). A masculine ideal that I call "companionate responsibility" has developed, characterized by domesticity, fidelity, and self-care, as well as responsible provision (Wentzell and Inhorn 2014). Living out this currently ideal form of modern masculinity amid the economic and social constraints of life today has become a key "moral project" for many Mexican men (Yarris and Ponting 2019: 39). This ideal bridges the provider aspects of prior ideals for husbands and fathers with the emphasis on emotional closeness central to companionate marriage. It is highly visible in Cuernavaca. For instance, local antiviolence protests have been led by a model of engaged fathering: the poet Javier Sicilia, who began to organize in response to his son's murder (Padgett 2011). As in other Mexican cities, people's responses to violence often include critiques of "traditional" masculinities, from criticism of *violencia machista* (macho violence) to attempts to reform men but maintain patriarchal structures among the growing population of evangelical Christians in the city (Brito 2016; Haney 2012).

Companionate marriage and responsibility were what Arturo sought to better embody when he promised God that he would improve as a husband and father. Our interviews served as one of many daily life sites for he and Ade to engage in emotional intimacy. They were physically demonstrative and emotionally engaged as we talked—quick to laugh together and to touch the other's leg or hand when discussing difficult times. They had valued emotional connection from the start, telling me that from the time they met as teenagers, each had been attracted to the other's kindness and the ways their partner helped others. For instance, Arturo said that Ade "doesn't know how to be harsh" and "helps almost everyone," counting off a list of the neighbors, friends, and coworkers she had supported. She saw his dedication to his church peers and the HIM study as similarly valuable. They also agreed that they had, in his words, "matured" together during their twenty-six-year relationship. Ade attributed this to deliberate, joint engagement in self-improvement. She said, "We've grown a lot together. Each of us on our own has taken courses in humanism, personal advancement, psychology." She added that Arturo's religious conversion "has really nurtured his life, his character, his behavior. Although he was always kind, calm, caring, attentive, home-bodied—that increased." Laughing, she said that she herself used to be more controlling and quick to anger but had calmed in response to Arturo's changes: "If he didn't explode, well, I didn't either, since I didn't have anyone to yell at." He said that over time they have changed as a couple and as parents, becoming more tolerant and trusting of family members' desires and interests. This emphasis on shared emotional growth lies at the heart of contemporary Mexico's companionate ideals.

Cuernavaca was an ideal site for this study since, beyond housing the HIM study, the city is a microcosm of many of the key social histories, changes, and problems facing Mexico. The capital of Morelos State, located eighty-five kilometers south of Mexico City, Cuernavaca is a former elite vacation site where colonizers' summer palaces now serve as tourist attractions. For decades the city has experienced rapid growth marked by economic inequality (Aguayo Quezada et al. 2014). The metropolitan area now contains more than 900,000 people (Consejo Estatal de Población de Morelos 2013). This includes a diversity of largely mestizo-identified residents: affluent bedroom communities of Mexico City workers, families who migrated in the 1960s to work in emerging industrial zones, and residents of once-rural towns absorbed in the sprawl. Cuernavaca's poverty rate is low relative to the rest of the nation yet still painfully high at 26.5 percent, with the vast majority of the population identified as vulnerable to economic want or deprivation of social services (CONEVAL 2012).

The once-peaceful metropolitan area has also entered a dramatic security crisis. Over time the violence that represents the "dark side" of maintaining a stable yet corrupt federal government has affected new areas of the country (Pansters 2012: 8). Fallout from the intensification of the federal drug war of the early 2000s destabilized the established patterns of corruption and criminal turf control that had meant safety for everyday people in Cuernavaca (Knight 2012; Melgar Bao 2005). In 2009, a cartel turf war generated a crime wave that eventually led the metro area to become one of the highest-crime sites in the country (Miranda 2012; Pastrana 2011; Seguridad 2012, 2015). Rates of extortion, violent robbery, and kidnapping for ransom have skyrocketed since the mid-2000s (Aguayo Quezada et al. 2014; Seguridad 2015).

This insecurity has been intensified by a feedback loop between criminal violence and the ravages of the global economic crisis. Together, these factors sharply curtailed the construction and tourism jobs that had been critical to the local economy. In a local version of a growing national trend, the formerly ubiquitous crowds of American college students studying Spanish in Cuernavaca have disappeared from the streets. (See also Luna 2018 for a borderlands example.) This situation is worsened by the fact that the zone's youthful population, with about half of residents age twenty-nine or younger, is suffering from lack of employment and educational opportunity (Peña González 2014). As on the national level, in Cuernavaca political corruption has precluded an effective response to these linked violence and economic crises. Morelos State was recently rated as the second most corrupt in the nation in a national assessment (Aguayo Quezada et al. 2014). As a result, almost no Cuernavacans say they trust public institutions such as the police force (Peña González 2014).

Arturo's carjacking made him one of many victims of this situation. His response of religious conversion also appears to be common. Evangelical Christianities, locally glossed as *Cristianismo*, are increasingly visible in Cuernavaca. For example, one congregation built the city's first American-style megachurch during my research for this book. While statistics are not available to indicate whether conversion has increased in response to recent insecurity, discourses about conversion in Cuernavaca reflect ongoing critiques of machismo, economic inequality, and violence, offering religious practice as a way to counteract and heal from social problems.

While they express it in diverse actions that range from religious to medical practice, Cuernavacans of all social classes report changing their behavior in response to the rising crime (cf. Tonantzin 2013). Surveys show that the majority of residents have curtailed daily life activities such as going out at night, going out alone, and using public transportation (Aguayo Quezada et al. 2014). People have also become despairing of the notion that collective solutions might arise. Although activism is visible in the city—for example, in marches organized by the Catholic Church against government corruption and violence (*La Redacción* 2016)—few people think that those in their neighborhood or community would organize to address political, social, or health problems (Aguayo Quezada et al. 2014). Instead, like others faced with navigating the "routinization of violence" in Latin America (Davis 2018), people have attempted to adapt their behavior to survive these new and frightening circumstances. This book explores how people have incorporated their involvement in the HIM study into such responses, showing that even as people lose hope in government aid or collective action, they still hope to heal the collective through their *own* actions. Beyond simply trying to stay safe, HIM participants often came to see the study as a way to live out and promote responsible, caring, and modern behavior that they hoped would provide a counterpoint to the societal dissolution happening around them, and thus help to heal the social body.

Cuernavaca's health services infrastructure figured into these hopes. While people voiced disgust for politicians, they also believed the government should live up to postrevolutionary promises of care for the people. These promises were reflected in the city's public universities, research centers, and hospitals from which people sought services even as they dismissed other areas of the government, such as the police and judiciary. The HIM study was based in the regional hospital of the IMSS, a federal entity that offers free health care to all privately employed workers as one of many projects intended to foster modern, healthy mestizo families. Many of its workers and patients became HIM participants, seeking to further the system's goals in both their research participation and daily lives. For instance, as an IMSS nurse, Ade believed that she was duty-bound to promote comprehensive visions of health within and beyond her formal job requirements. Frustrated by the cursory sexual health education she saw her daughters receive as teens, she took training as a sexual educator and sought information about HPV from the HIM staff. Hoping to "plant a seed . . . to prevent a little," Ade gave formal talks at schools and used the brief breaks in her busy IMSS workdays to waylay teens waiting for medical services and "offer them information about prevention," such as condom use.

The fact that there are teens waiting for hours at the IMSS clinic demonstrates another key aspect of the public health system: in Cuernavaca and elsewhere, its goals are undercut by underfunding and government unreliability. The IMSS and other social security organizations reflect a history of governments that have ruled by selectively providing services amid widespread corruption. While the postrevolutionary Mexican state has always faced challenges from both disenfranchised groups and organized crime, it has maintained greater stability than many other Latin American countries by coupling repression and criminal alliances with very real (if unequally distributed) efforts to provide health and social services in keeping with citizens' constitutionally mandated rights (Knight 1992; Matsuura 2013). Megan Crowley-Matoka (2016) calls Mexico a "slippery State," in which citizens expect aid but cannot predict, in any particular interaction, whether they will meet with competence or corruption, disorganization or resource scarcity. She describes state institutions as "widely understood to be at once a source of vital resources (such as health care) *and* profoundly corrupt" (Crowley-Matoka 2016: 126). The IMSS itself is both credited with a major role in increasing the population's life expectancy and critiqued for chronic underfunding and uneven quality and availability of services (Moreno et al. 2009; Notimex 2014).

Yet while Mexican citizens overwhelmingly view politicians and government institutions as corrupt and ineffectual, they tend to call not for privatized alternatives but for a rehabilitated state to meet its mandate of caring for its citizens. Citizens have previously responded to state failures to provide reliable protection and care by protesting and by forming community organizations to offer the services that the state promotes but often fails to provide (Schneider 2010). Today, IMSS workers and beneficiaries are actively protesting against recent government reforms that incorporate elements of privatization (see, e.g., Lopez 2015). Overall, beneficiaries tend to see the IMSS as an imperiled but important vestige of a revolutionary federal commitment to the public good, which might not be reliably efficient or trustworthy but should be bolstered rather than dismantled (Crowley-Matoka and Lock 2006).

Simultaneous commitment to the IMSS and its goals, and frustration about the availability of its services, influenced many people's decisions to participate in the HIM study. This was the case for Arturo and Ade, who learned about HIM through Ade's IMSS job; they believed the study was trustworthy because of its association with the IMSS, but they also enrolled Arturo in part to access more responsive health services. Ade noted that as an IMSS worker she could get medical testing whenever she needed by using her social connections in the hospital. Yet while Arturo had access to cost-free IMSS care, to use it he would have to face what Ade described as the "lines and lines and lines of people" always waiting. They saw his HIM participation as providing more responsive first-line care because, as Ade noted, "It's a complete study," as well as the only local site where men could be tested for HPV. Arturo saw his clinical visits as "practical, quick and secure." Further, the intimate testing was done with "so much trustworthiness, so much hygiene and so much ethical commitment" that Arturo felt confident letting HIM staff "enter in [his] intimate zone" without "feeling intimidated or ashamed." For many men, participation in this research program that was in, but not of, the IMSS gave them access to the care they felt they were owed by the state in a more timely and reliable way. They were so pleased with the attentive care and range of tests that they often characterized their visits as providing a thorough checkup, despite the testing's actual focus on sexual health issues.

THE HIM STUDY AND POPULATION

The HIM study is a multinational investigation of the "natural history" of HPV in men. Human papillomavirus is actually a family of viruses; some can cause warts and others can cause pre-cancerous or cancerous lesions, which can affect many areas of the body. Genital HPV strains are collectively considered the world's most common sexually transmitted infection (STI). While most people who contract HPV never experience symptoms (although they can transmit the virus while it is active), some infections lead to genital warts or cancers of the cervix, penis, anus, head, and neck (Clifford et al. 2005). Since cervical cancer is by far the most common HPV-related cancer, and since women's sexual and reproductive health is under far more scrutiny than men's, HPV is often seen as a women's concern. The HIM study aims to shed light on men's epidemiological experience of HPV, since men are as likely to contract and transmit it as women, but little is known about this phenomenon.

The HIM study is funded by the U.S. National Institutes of Health but has an international scope, with sites in the United States, Brazil, and Mexico. The study aimed to establish a group of three thousand men who would be tested for HPV every six months for four years to shed light on how the virus develops and clears in men and better understand the health and behavioral factors that lead some infections to clear and others to persist or become symptomatic (Giuliano et al. 2006). Enrollment began in 2005, and testing continued long afterward as the study found additional grant support. The study was a longitudinal and observational study, which means that it monitored participants' biological changes over a long time span rather than testing a health intervention. This makes it a different setting from the shorter-term, intervention-based clinical trials on which much social-science research has focused. Because of its long-term influence on participants' daily lives, and the reflection on their behavior and biological changes that it can generate, longitudinal, observational research is an ideal setting for investigating how people incorporate medical research participation into their broader, ongoing efforts to be particular kinds of people and cope with specific social changes.

Participants in the HIM study were tested with new DNA technology that reveals previously undetectable asymptomatic HPV infection. At each visit, participants also completed computerized surveys regarding their health and sexual practices and received written records of their prior STI test results. At the Cuernavaca site, participants did a circuit of tests, moving among the various stations set up in the research clinic. They gave a urine sample in the bathroom, had blood drawn at the phlebotomy station, sat at the computer carrel to complete the questionnaires, then entered a private cubicle with the physician's desk and an exam bed for their HPV testing.

Given the length of the study, participants and staff got to know one another well over time; the staff also prided themselves on being friendly and open to encourage participants to keep returning. As participants moved through the tests, they would chat with staff about their families and children, providing life updates about the previous six months. The two physicians, one male and one female, who did the genital testing also had cordial relationships with the participants. They would catch up, although, as the female physician noted, "total silence" fell once men sat on the exam table. For genital testing, men were asked to strip below the waist and lie on a bed. The doctor would observe the men's genitals for signs of sexually transmitted infection, then rub cotton swabs along their penis and scrotum (as well as their anus for those men who consented). If necessary, they would also offer STI-related medical treatment, such as the removal of genital warts. After the genital exam, the participant (and his wife, if she had accompanied him) would sit in an office with the physician or clinical director to receive an explanation of the STI testing results from the participant's last visit. Men were given a slip of paper that stated whether they were negative or positive for "low-risk" (potentially wart-causing) or "high-risk" (potentially cancer-causing) HPV strains. The staff member would explain the possible consequences of the diagnosis, suggest that wives of high-risk positive men be screened for cervical cancer, and answer questions.

The study was run by a Cuernavaca-based public health research unit of the IMSS. Thus, it was based in the IMSS offices—first, in the regional IMSS hospital, then across the street, and finally in the purpose-built research clinic in the city center that had been under construction since the inception of my research. These sites were sunny and clean and decorated with research posters from the unit's other projects, which connoted a privileged position in the IMSS hierarchy and framed the office as a site of successful knowledge generation. These IMSS connections were crucial to study recruitment. The study recruited heavily within the IMSS staff and patient populations, as well as at local universities and large businesses with IMSS-eligible staff (Giuliano et al. 2006). It is illegal to pay medical research participants in Mexico, so Mexican HIM participants were uncompensated aside from free STI treatment and a few courtesy medical tests (including cholesterol and bone density testing) offered to them and their spouses. Thus, recruitment focused on the individual and societal benefits of participation. The HIM staff gave talks discussing HPV, related cancers, and the fact that men can have and transmit the virus. They called on men to aid in the research endeavor and noted that the HIM study was the only way for men to get HPV testing. Many participants recounted that their own or their wives' attendance at one of these talks was their impetus for joining the study.

The staff also used posters, placed throughout IMSS clinical buildings, to recruit men by framing participation as a way to support others and perform modern and responsible masculinity and fatherhood. For instance, one poster combined images of men, boys, and infants to call on men as fathers to aid in prevention efforts. Another showed the respectable and proud-looking male HIM staff members, together with an image of men's raised fists, with the wording "Together for Men's Health"; the heading "You Can Help by Participating in This Important Study" was superimposed over the backdrop of the IMSS regional hospital. This sent the message that men could enact companionate responsibility while supporting and benefiting from government care.

This kind of framing appealed to a specific group of men who tended already to be working to support public health and seeking to live out what they saw as modern masculinities. Overall, while formal HIM inclusion criteria focused on the absence of an active STI, the Cuernavaca HIM population also had a higher level of formally employed, highly educated, and relatively economically stable participants with access to state health care than the population at large. The reason was that participants recruited at the IMSS and private companies were usually formally employed, a status that provides relative economic stability (though not necessarily wealth) in a country where most people work in the informal economy (INEGI 2009). Many participants and their spouses were state workers, mostly in the IMSS, but also in education and scientific research.

The subset of this group who participated in my research were likely especially predisposed to relate medical research participation to broader life projects, including those involving the sorts of care on which many focused professionally in state health and education jobs. As I discuss further in the appendix, HIM staff recruited for my study and selected participants they thought would be willing to participate. This meant inviting those who seemed especially invested in HIM participation, had demonstrated an interest and willingness in talking about their broader lives and the HIM study's place within it in informal conversations during medical procedures, and reliably showed up to appointments. It was fairly common for participants in my study to say that they were interested in doing our interviews because they believed in the merit of research generally, wished to support the IMSS and IMSS-allied initiatives that could help others, and found meaning in talking about their life experiences. This population was thus a subset of a subset. They were probably not representative of all Cuernavaca HIM participants, some of whom might have enrolled with primarily medical benefits or other ends in mind, or might have experienced HIM as a clinically bounded or generally unimportant experience. Their specific experiences are important to understand not because they are representative, but because they reveal how people can use medical research participation to further context-specific, extraclinical ends unanticipated by study designers.

For the anthropological study population, these contexts included the discourses on Mexicanness and gender and the experiences of the economic and violence crises, discussed earlier; they also included a specifically urban, middle-class take on long-standing local cultural ideologies regarding collectivity. People across demographics in Mexico often cite emphasis on familial closeness as both a fact of Mexican society and a matter of national pride (cf. Crowley-Matoka 2016). This emphasis is not limited to kin. For example, casting Mexican society as one "revolutionary family" served as a postrevolutionary political justification for single-party rule (Zolov 1999). Deliberately creating and expanding one's kinship networks has also been a feature of Mexican society since conquest. The system of *compradrazgo*—a form of ritual kinship in which parents select people to be their children's godparents, and thus their own coparents, as children go through Catholic life-course rituals— has served to create relationships of mutual aid and obligation (Carlos 1973).

While cultural emphasis on the family endures, what kinship looks like amid urbanization and cultural efforts at "modernization" has changed. For instance, forms of compradrazgo had already shifted in cities by the 1970s, with the creation of ties limited to only baptism rituals and more likely to be made with existing kin and people from one's socioeconomic stratum than powerful patrons (Carlos 1973). The rise of Mexican versions of globally emerging "middle-class" subjectivities also involved shifting conceptions of family. In Mexico, the emergence of this sort of middle class occurred amid both economic crisis and partial government efforts toward neoliberal governance and the related logic of capitalist individuality. Thus, middle-class subjectivities came to involve emphasis on personal development that could contribute to familial, rather than primarily individual, well-being in an uncertain world (Careaga Valdez 1987; Vieyra Bahena 2018). This process, in tandem with the idealization of companionate marriage and its emphasis on the marital dyad, led to a change in focus within the meaning of family for middle-class Mexicans, from a focus on extended kin networks to nuclear families (Ramirez and Everett 2018).

The HIM participants I interviewed overwhelmingly emphasized the importance of family in these terms, merging characteristically middle-class aspirations for personal development into efforts to enhance collective well-being, significantly, but not only, at the level of the family. This emphasis on leading others forward through self-care and development notably displaced emphases on mutual aid through systems such as compradrazgo. Although such ties remain key to social life in many Mexican contexts (see, e.g., Cant 2018), participants in my study never mentioned them at all.

Middle-class takes on family were also evident in relationship to participants' conceptions of health. The main contribution of this book is to highlight how people hoped men's participation in the HIM study would aid the biological, as well as social, well-being of others with whom they were related. Yet they focused these hopes on experiences with biomedicine, a healing system focused on individual patients. Valeria Napolitano (2002) argues that, in the pluralistic healing worlds of urban Mexico, people's choices of health intervention also reveal their ideas about how forms of sociality influence sickness. She notes that by choosing particular modalities, such as traditional Chinese medicine, people simultaneously cope with the local economic and other constraints on health-care access while aligning themselves with particular visions of modernity or cosmopolitanism (Napolitano and Mora Flores 2003). In this light, it is notable that HIM participants avoided the traditional healing practices that remain common in Mexico, even though these practices resonate with collective visions of health. Such practices often focus on relationships in ways that range from healing the physical consequences of relationships gone awry (in the case of witchcraft beliefs) and cleansing the energy of the homes and family of sick people (as sometimes occurs in the more mainstream versions of *curanderismo* commonly practiced). Aside from one participant who received a certification to teach traditional Mexican healing in a university setting, participants who used complementary forms of healing focused on imported systems that had a more elite cultural cachet. Some used traditional Chinese medicine, and several took and sold supplements such as Herbalife that fused scientific-sounding promises with logics of capitalist self-improvement. By reframing biomedicine as a health intervention that could act on relational problems, participants crafted distinctly middle-class takes on collectivity that fused culturally resonant emphases on family and relationality with the use of systems that signaled modernity and upward mobility. (For other examples of the emphasis on family relationships as central to patient care within Mexican biomedicine, see Crowley-Matoka 2016; Hale 2017.)

The Study Design

This book is based on a series of annual interviews with thirty-one heterosexual HIM participants and their female partners, comparison groups of ten men and twelve women interviewed without their spouses, and HIM staff.

In the appendix I discuss the study design and how I analyzed data. Briefly, I did the open-ended Spanish-language interviews from 2010 to 2013, with additional follow-up in 2015. My goal in focusing on couples rather than individuals was to center collective experience from the start to understand sexual health as an interpersonal rather than individual experience and to more easily identify the consequences of men's participation in medical research over time beyond their individual bodies. I focused specifically on heterosexual couples both because the vast majority of Mexican HIM participants had female primary partners and to understand how changing ideologies of heterosexual marriage had influenced couples' study experiences. I did not find significant thematic differences between the statements of couples interviewed together and individuals alone, with the exception of some people's willingness to tell me marital "secrets" individually that they did not wish to share in front of their spouses.

Focusing on interviews was the best way to study relationships between HIM participation and peoples' daily lives, given the particular constraints of a medical research study field site. Cultural anthropologists famously use participant observation in people's daily lives to gather diverse forms of data regarding what people do, which is rarely identical to what they say or think they do. Yet medical research studies—and anthropological studies of them—are required to guarantee participant confidentiality. This meant that I had to confine my research with HIM participants largely to the clinical setting. I was permitted to interact outside the HIM offices only with those participants who chose to invite me to do so; I could not ask for such invitations, as this might pressure participants to compromise confidentiality. Most who did so were evangelical Christians, so data from participant observation appears largely in chapter 6, where I discuss that group's experiences. In most participants' cases, interviews were the most feasible and appropriate method for me to understand how spouses collaborated to make sense of the interactions between their HIM and broader life experiences.

Both my conduct and analysis of these interviews were shaped by an "ethnographic sensibility," which the anthropologist Carole McGranahan (2018: 4) describes as a culturally rooted "commitment to interpersonal relations as the base of knowledge" reliant on insights from a researcher's long-term engagement with people and place. The interviews were designed to address topics I suspected from experience would be relevant for participants' understandings of HIM involvement and to enable participants to raise issues I had not anticipated. My goal in structuring the interviews was to encourage participants to guide the conversation to their own topics of interest, and for couples to talk together, so that I could learn about their interactive efforts to make meaning out of medical research experience in this particular social setting. As they did so, I paid attention to their nonverbal interactions and silences, as well as their narratives. I understand the resulting data to reveal peoples' joint and sometimes interpersonally fraught efforts to be particular kinds of people in research-related settings. Since people are likely to be strategically vague about potentially stigmatizing sexual issues in daily life but more open about them in medical settings (Carillo 2002; Finkler 1991), these interviews provided a unique space for such efforts.

I analyze the content of these interviews not as a journalistic reflection of experience, but as context-specific presentations of self that people created in collaboration with all those present (Jackson 1998; Linde 1993). This includes myself. The fact that I am a woman likely facilitated men's discussion of vulnerabilities and women's discussions of their experiences, but it also probably precluded specific presentations of self such as more "traditional" masculinities (González-López 2005; Hirsch 2003; Hirsch et al. 2007). My U.S. nationality likely encouraged participants to speak of themselves "as Mexicans" and seek to educate me on what they thought that meant. Participants expressed strong and contradictory views of the United States, describing it as simultaneously aspirationally modern and wealthy and a driver of racialized economic inequality in the region. They understood me, as a white American, as representing both of these aspects. Thus, I became an audience for critiques of U.S. culture and dominance, as well as an interlocutor understood as sympathetic to modernizing projects, including those with implicit goals of population whitening. My status as a researcher amplified the latter feelings of kinship, with participants in medical and academic careers understanding me to be from a similar work milieu and to hold shared goals for aiding society through our labor.

Any research methodology opens a window onto the issue under study, revealing that which is visible from a particular angle and vantage point (Haraway 1988). In this study, interviews revealed people's context-specific reflections about physical and social interactions, as well as spouses' collaborative efforts to make narrative sense of them. While inherently partial, the view presented here reveals key and little-known ways that people can incorporate ostensibly individual medical research participation into efforts to affect their and others' lives and bodies beyond the clinic.

In the chapters that follow, I show how HIM participants and their partners incorporated the medical research experience into efforts to care for social bodies and heal the collective biologies to which they belonged. I analyze their narratives of research participation to reveal how they hoped this activity would be useful at multiple levels of scale.

Chapter 2 initiates the analysis of HIM participants' experiences at multiple levels of scale by exploring men's personal experiences of gendered selfhood and change. I discuss men's efforts to incorporate medical research involvement into performances of companionate responsibility, done in collaboration with their wives and in relationship to enduring ideologies of machismo. The chapter thus shows the "individual" level of gendered self-hood to be fundamentally relational, in context-specific ways. In chapter 3 I explore how the gender ideology participants articulated in chapter 2 in-fluences their understandings of HPV biology, transmission, and the social risks it could pose. I show that spouses drew on local ideologies of collective biology to frame men's individual HPV testing as a way to monitor and en-hance the health of their shared "couples biology." In chapter 4 I discuss how couples' HIM participation reflected and enhanced their ability to be good parents—for example, by ensuring they would be healthy enough to support their children and enabling them to model health-promoting gender and marital practices for them. In chapter 5 I investigate how participants and partners also hoped to advance the Mexican social body as a whole through such modeling. This analysis shows how they sought to advance the nation by embodying and promoting a "culture of prevention" related to non-macho masculinities and companionate marriage. In this way, HIM participation came to serve as a form of citizenship though which couples supported the spirit of national public health programs and strove to guide the Mexican populace forward, despite rising violence and the unreliability of their slip-pery state. Chapter 6 focuses on evangelical Christian participants' experi-ences. I discuss their incorporation of the HIM study into pious efforts to embody and model the health, gender, and marital practices their churches promoted. This adds complexity to the prior chapters' analysis of partici-pants' use of a local ideology of collective biology to understand HIM par-ticipation by demonstrating how people draw on multiple ways of under-standing the world to make sense of such pursuits. In chapter 7, I conclude the book by discussing the utility of the collective biologies approach for investigating relationships between individual behavior and the well-being of broader, nonindividual bodies. I suggest ways that this approach can be used in medical research, its ethics oversight, and public health practice.

Through this inquiry I show that seemingly individual health behavior can have embodied social consequences that extend widely beyond the clinic and the individual body. My findings broaden our understanding of this phenomenon in medical research, since social-science study of that field has focused on resource-poor or marginalized participants seeking care or social inclusion through short-term global clinical trials that test medical interventions (see, e.g., Elliott and Abadie 2008; Geissler 2015; Nguyen 2009; Petryna 2009). These findings also shed light on the understudied role that gender plays in people's medical research experiences.

Beyond the case of medical research, the present study reveals how middle-class people incorporate long-term health surveillance into ongoing daily life efforts to be good and modern people, partners, parents, and citizens. The findings discussed here are specific to the Mexican context, where mestizos have long been encouraged to view their health practices as ways to set themselves apart from Indigenous or impoverished others. They are also influenced by the violence crisis that struck Cuernavaca during the study, to which they responded by framing HIM participation as a way to help others and contribute to national health and modernization at a time of instability. Yet I use these specific insights to make a broader point: that attending to multiple levels of scale when assessing medical research participation, health surveillance, or, indeed, any health behavior is necessary for understanding how people draw on local cultural currents and events to assess the embodied consequences of their actions.

I hope that the analysis in the coming chapters can model a way of identifying and assessing the complexly biosocial interrelationships between individual behavior and the well-being of the particular nonindividual bodies that exist in specific cultural settings. I offer the analytic of collective biologies as a way to operationalize this study of relationships among bodies on multiple levels of scale. This book is a study of how people can collaborate to use seemingly individual health practices to treat collective ills. In it, I aim to model an approach that could also be useful for understanding this phenomenon in diverse cultural contexts, and beyond social-science inquiry in medical research design, ethics oversight, and public health practice. I also hope this analysis will model a way of assessing how people can draw on collective ideologies in responses to pressing problems, despite globally increasing political and economic pressures toward individualization.

TWO

PERFORMING MODERN MASCULINITIES
IN MEDICAL RESEARCH

Mario, a fifty-year-old bartender, told me that he enrolled in the HIM study "for my wife, who suggested it, and because really here in Mexico we're a bit macho, but you have to move beyond that, little by little, participating in health projects." Mario's explanation connected his personal experience with medical research participation directly to relationships beyond the clinic. He was inspired to enroll by his relationship with his wife Paty, a nurse with the Instituto Mexicano del Seguro Social (IMSS) who heard about the study at work. He then interpreted his experiences with the Human Papillomavirus in Men (HIM) study in light of his relationship to the category of Mexican men, who he understood as prone to machismo but able to move beyond it through progressive practices. Mario noted, "It's important to me not to be macho," and recounted being taught by his father from childhood that "in the house there weren't machos. There were sons, a family, and that everyone had to work equally."

Despite his lifelong effort to engage in egalitarian practices of gender, Mario discussed the fear that innately macho tendencies lurked within him

due to his nature as a Mexican man. He explicitly used HIM study procedures as opportunities to identify and then challenge such tendencies. For
example, he said that the anogenital swabbing required for human papillomavirus (HPV) testing "at the start made me a little reluctant, because here
in Mexico, the machismo is really high and, well, they take samples from
parts that they normally don't from a man." He then reported deliberately
working through this reluctance, including by inviting Paty to accompany
him to clinical appointments and thus embracing emotionally engaged marriage as an antidote to traditionally gendered shame.

Mario further hoped to use his medical research experience to model
difference from machismo for others. Seeking to foster change in Mexican
masculinities on a generational timeline, he hoped that his sons would
learn from his efforts. He explained, "Normally here [in Mexico] a man
finds it very difficult to let someone touch his intimate parts, and, well, I
got accustomed to it. Now I see it as something normal. . . . We're transmitting all that to our sons." He and Paty also hoped that he could lead
the populace as a whole by example, since, she complained, "Usually in a
clinic waiting room it's women and children. . . . Rarely do you see men."
Mario thus collaborated with Paty to understand his HIM experiences
within collective experiences of family and nation and to hope those experiences would contribute to positive change over time within those biosocial
bodies.

In this chapter, I discuss how men such as Mario incorporated HIM participation into their individual efforts to live out desired masculinities. Such
efforts frequently revolved around the concept of machismo. People in
Mexico often frame machismo as a shared trait that good men must struggle against to better embody modernity and the privileged racial and class
categories associated with modern behavior. Researchers have found this
logic to underlie men's efforts to make changes that include quitting drinking, infidelity, and violence (Amuchástegui Herrera 2008; Brandes 2002;
Wentzell 2013).

Here I examine how participants understood their HIM experiences in this
way. While I never introduced the concept of machismo in our interviews,
participants often did. They incorporated their HIM study experiences into
their narratives of efforts to continue being "different" from regressively macho
Mexican men in the abstract, or to adopt such difference over time. Here I
discuss how participants used specific study experiences, such as repeated
testing for sexually transmitted infections (STIs), as tools for demonstrating

modern health behavior or thwarting desires to act in macho ways that they viewed as innate but problematic.

Since men such as Mario understood their intimate clinical experiences to affect broader collectives to which they belonged—from the family to the Mexican populace—I aim to honor their perspective by keeping relationships in the analytic frame even as I focus on men's narratives of their personal and often internal experience. This approach makes sense since gender is an inherently relational practice (Butler 1990; Gutmann 2007). It is particularly necessary in a context where people so vocally discuss masculinities as both deriving from the historical relationships that created mestizaje, and as changing or enduring on the societal level in relationship to individual men's abilities to engage in behavior cast as modern rather than macho (Amuchástegui and Szasz 2007; Gutmann 1996).

This explicit emphasis on relationships is also central to emerging Mexican cultural ideals of masculinity framed in opposition to machismo. Many participants expressly rejected machismo in ways that enabled them to live out an emerging masculine ideal that I call "companionate responsibility" (Wentzell and Inhorn 2014). This is the globally emergent idea that good, modern men should provide emotionally as well as materially through intimate and faithful engagement with wives and children (cf. Heron 2019). Cuernavacan participants' takes on companionate responsibility reflected their specific context. The populace was suffering from narcoviolence attributed to hard-hearted men who valued wealth over life; people protesting against this violence often called for or modeled engaged fathering and anti-macho masculinities (see, e.g., Padgett 2011).

So in this chapter I examine how men asserted and reconfigured specific forms of gendered selfhood through their HIM experiences. I frame men's intimate, lived experience of masculinity as the smallest level of scale in the interacting, variously sized set of biosocial bodies that subsequent chapters explore. To do this, I focus on men's discussions of their own internal experiences of activities such as HPV testing and their narratives of how such experiences demonstrated existing or facilitated desired difference from "typical" Mexican manhood. Given the profoundly relational nature of their narratives of these events, I include participants' perceptions of others, and the voices of wives who deeply influenced participants' ways of being men, to faithfully portray men's experiences of performing masculinities through medical research participation.

Research Participation as an Anti-macho Act

Many men saw the health surveillance and intimate anogenital testing that HIM participation required as evidence that they were rejecting macho masculinity in their daily lives. This was the case for Davíd, an IMSS clerical worker in his early thirties. Davíd cast his participation as a mark of his difference from typical Mexican men, which, together with a general interest in health and love of reading, demonstrated his "open mind." He attributed a "lack of culture" to abstract Mexican men, which, he believed, deterred them from seeking health care. He noted, "In our culture it's not a given that the Mexican man understands health, because there's a lot of machismo." Davíd's HIM participation appeared to be a way to demonstrate his progressive difference by showing that he "like[s] to study the body, to pay attention to health." This intellectual interest served as a marker of his education and higher class status.

It also demonstrated his commitment to companionate responsibility, since Davíd discussed his health not as an individual issue, but as a resource that would help him care for his wife and family. For example, he said he avoided infidelity "for fear of getting my wife sick." Self-care, including HIM participation, was a way to demonstrate that although "we [Mexican men] are really careless, . . . I consider myself responsible." His individual HIM enrollment thus enabled him to define himself as a good man within his relationships to his wife and to the category of Mexican men in the abstract.

Such claims that HIM participation represented positive and protective difference from abstract others were common. For instance, Benjamín, a taxicab driver, explained his decision to enroll in terms of such difference: "There aren't people like us, who want to discover, really understand, what they have, right?" This sense of having an uncommon commitment to positive personal development influenced his and his wife's practices of parenting, as well. I discuss their efforts to care for their family through positive role modeling of health-care participation and other self-consciously modern traits in chapter 4.

Several men identified not only HIM enrollment but also the lived experience of HPV testing as something that made them different from abstract, macho Mexican men. They often discussed the physical experience of HPV testing as one of vulnerability. They noted, sometimes implicitly and sometimes explicitly, that their research participation entailed procedures that a stereotypically macho man would find emasculating. This was because more traditional frameworks of masculinity in Mexico attributed manliness to being the one who penetrates others and, more broadly, puts others in physically and sexually vulnerable positions (Melhuus 1998). Undergoing penile and, especially, anal swabbing in the social position of subordination to the physician in a medical encounter could be interpreted as akin to feminizing penetration. Recognizing this possibility, the lab tech Raúl said that during rectal examination, "I don't feel any shame. I'm used to it. It never stops being uncomfortable, but health comes first. At the [IMSS], I've heard lots of people with a problem, who've had it for twenty years. They never went to the doctor because of shame, even shame of being seen naked. They just don't get treatment, and the problems get worse." Raúl contrasted himself with those who followed the macho line that their bodies were invulnerable and were thus unwilling to open themselves up to medical scrutiny. Instead, he cast his own openness to health testing—and bravery despite discomfort—as manly attributes.

Like Raúl, participants employed in the health field were especially likely to frame their acceptance of intimate testing as evidence of both good masculinity and higher class, educational, and implicitly racial status than macho others. For instance, Leo, a clerical worker at the IMSS, said that undergoing the tests was not difficult, "because I work in a hospital, too. They were hard at the start, but by the second time, normal. Like checking your throat or eyes. That's the doctor's job. It's a study that helps us." Similarly, Pablo, a physician, said the sampling was easy because he was "used to medical studies. That's the medical culture. They have to touch you, test you. It's not strange."

Many men discussed working through their initial discomfort with anogenital testing as evidence that they were actively rejecting the machismo they had inherited as Mexican men. For example, I asked Javier, a driver, whether the testing had been hard for him. "Yes, unfortunately our gender can be a little macho," he responded. "I'm not used to being touched like that, so there's a little shame, embarrassment." However, he said that since the study physicians were respectful and he believed the testing was worthwhile, he had overcome the discomfort and now saw the testing as "not a big deal." Adalberto, a factory manager, had reached a similar place. He recounted, "The personal samples—at first they're tough. They tell you to take off your pants, and where they'll touch you, and you feel a little shame. But it's worth it to feel secure, for me and my wife." He explicitly framed the care the testing provided for the couple's interrelated biology as the worthwhile outcome of embarrassing testing. His willingness to get over that shame to access couple's care was thus evidence of his successful performance of companionate responsibility. Pedro, a taxicab driver, also appeared to think the collective benefits of HPV testing outweighed the potential threat they posed to masculinity. He linked HPV surveillance to being a good father with the comment that getting testing was "what I had to do, to help my kids." I discuss Pedro's and others' hopes for such collective benefits further in subsequent chapters.

Several participants talked about the experience of being tested by a female physician as a particular challenge for demonstrating anti-macho attitudes. For instance, the retired accountant Ricardo said, "It does give me a little shame when it's a woman doctor. But you get used to it." This was also true for the dental technician Rafael, who said he came to see this as "embarrassing but necessary" and to believe that "you have to adapt to that being normal to obtain the results." He remarked, "Those things aren't very normal in our culture," but asserted that Mexican culture would have to change, as it had when women became accustomed to pap tests to promote health and well-being. By making such changes in himself, Rafael explicitly hoped to be part of a broader change for good in a society he characterized as increasingly "more aggressive and less tolerant." For instance, he critiqued the machismo he viewed as transmitted through regressive parenting, noting, "There are boys who from childhood grow up with that mentality, and it's because the father is violent, is aggressive—the mother, too—they go to soccer games and yell insults." Accepting intimate medical testing, especially from a female doctor, was a way to model difference from those problematic attitudes.

Not all men were able to accept a woman doing intimate testing or agreed to undergo anal swabbing (which they could refuse and still participate in the study through genital skin swabbing alone). Jaime, an IMSS lab technician, attributed his discomfort with those experiences to cultural mores. Regarding penile sampling, he said, "Everything was fine until one time I had a female doctor. That was hard, because I think that we're not used to, or we don't have the culture of, being treated by a woman, right? Even though it was a professional situation, we're still not accustomed to it. It's the shame, right?" Rather than claiming that having intimate testing done by a woman was objectively inappropriate or emasculating, Jaime somewhat shamefully attributed his feelings to the culture that he believed the shared "we" of Mexican men harbored, despite its poor fit with modern and professional medical practice. Jaime declined anal sampling for the same reason. He explained,

I didn't want them to take samples from there because I felt like it violated my space. It's an intimate thing, right? Or maybe, I don't know, it's a man thing. Yeah, because aside from that, we also lack the culture of getting checkups. . . . There's the idea that the man is the man, and they shouldn't touch you there because if they do, you stop being a man. You have that mentality and you say "Why would you touch me there?" So maybe it's that. It really takes us work.

Jaime attributed his discomfort to macho cultural beliefs that manliness was defined by being physically invulnerable and a sexual penetrator rather than a vulnerable penetratee (Melhuus 1998). However, he also criticized this view, identifying it as a barrier to health care that required work to get over rather than as a statement of fact to be accepted. Further linking his own experience to the broader population of Mexican men to which he attributed his cultural views of masculinity, he reminded me that he was not the only one to reject anal testing. He said, "I know other colleagues who also didn't want to do that part of the study for the same reasons, because, well, it takes work to disconnect with that part of the culture that tells us not to do it."

Despite his adherence to some macho tropes, Jaime, like other HIM participants, saw his willingness to participate in the penile sampling—and thus grapple with his own performance of entrenched cultural norms—to be a marker of his modernity. When I asked him why he continued in the study despite feeling this shame, he replied, "I'm a lab tech, so we're used to taking blood, vaginal swabs, urethral swabs, so I have a more open idea. I consider these studies normal. If you don't know, it's like they're insulting your dignity. Your space—it's very personal. That's the difference." Thus, he portrayed himself as a modern, well-educated man sufficiently versed in science and health care to value medical testing, albeit one still struggling against the innate machismo that made anal testing a threat to his masculinity as traditionally defined.

In addition to referencing the older cultural idea of real men as penetrators rather than penetratees as a reason that intimate sampling could feel emasculating, HIM participants and their partners sometimes noted that those procedures could feel feminizing because it was women who usually underwent genital procedures, such as pap smears. Men simply were not used to this kind of experience, while their female partners were. Some men incorporated this disparity into their efforts to live out companionate responsibility by accepting the anogenital testing. For instance, Adalberto said that he valued his ability to participate in the study, although every time study staff called to schedule an appointment, he thought, "Fuck, I have to do it again! It's uncomfortable, to drop your pants. But it's worth it." He added that part of this value lay in his increased ability to empathize with his wife's experience. He said, "I now understand what my wife goes through when she has [fertility] tests much better. She said, 'You have no idea what it's like,' and now I do." Thus, some men felt that the experience of intimate testing offered embodied knowledge that brought them closer to their wives.

Testing Facilitates Companionate Responsibility

In these examples, participants framed HIM study participation as one of many daily life practices through which they lived out male companionate responsibility more broadly. Yet doing this was not always easy for men who felt torn between desires to act out progressive masculinities and what they experienced as a shared cultural history of and biological predisposition to equate manliness with machismo. Some of those men said that the HIM experience itself served as an aid for performing non-macho behavior.

The frequent STI testing they underwent provided a sense of accountability that encouraged them to be mindful of sexual health and to remember that their sexual behavior would affect the couple's biology. This was the case for the IMSS clerical worker Francisco, who responded to his negative HPV tests by recommitting to fidelity. When asked whether the study affected his life, he said, "Yes, because I was negative. I thought, 'Good, I'll keep sticking to one partner.' You see the consequences that having many partners could have. It's better to be safe. All the tests are negative, so it's better that I keep myself that way." The IMSS lab technician José Luis felt similarly. He noted that this knowledge, and the responsibility he felt to disclose it, kept him faithful. He explained, "It limits me, knowing what I have. I couldn't have sex with a woman. I would have to say that I'm a carrier." With an eye to public health, he also noted that he did not want to "share the virus" through extramarital sex.

Marco, a factory worker, believed that frequent STI testing highlighted the health risks of extramarital sex for male participants. He explained, "We start to think a little more, right? Of the risk one runs if you want to have a little affair—well, now you know that that can come with a surprise [of an STI]. It makes one stop and think more." Such emphases on the broader health and social consequences that extramarital sex could have for the couple reflected the care for female partners that is a hallmark of companionate responsibility. These participants' statements also reflected the discourse that machismo was an innately Mexican male trait that led men toward infidelity and framed HIM participation as an aid for deliberately choosing to reject that tendency in favor of faithful, companionate responsibility. The

HPV testing helped some men stick to their goal of acting out what they saw as modern masculinity.

Incorporating the HIM Study into Male Change over Time

While some men saw companionate responsibility as fundamental to their characters throughout their lives, other HIM participants adopted it after a lengthy process of change away from macho behavior. Narratives of men changing their forms of masculinity over time, such as the one with which this book opened, are common in Cuernavaca. As ideals of what counts as good and manly behavior have changed over the past decades, many individual men have lived out similar shifts in their own lives, identifying with more macho beliefs when younger and more companionately responsible ways of being men as they have aged. For example, in my earlier research with older Cuernavacan men experiencing erectile difficulty I found that men commonly thought of themselves as maturing with age. They saw their decreased ability to have penetrative sex not as a health problem, but as a respite from the innate machismo that they believed had led them to be unfaithful in younger years. They believed this change enabled them to be more modern, domestically oriented husbands and grandfathers in later life (Wentzell 2013). Such narratives of change over time were also common among the next generation largely represented here, as reflected in the ways that some couples discussed medical research participation as marking or facilitating manly change.

ALBERTO AND VERO: HIM PARTICIPATION
REFLECTS GENDERED CHANGE

Take, for example, the IMSS driver Alberto and his wife, Vero, a homemaker and shoe vendor. They had engaged in a lengthy process of marital change several years before he enrolled in the HIM study. The physically demonstrative, upbeat couple collaborated in our interviews on a shared narrative of deliberate masculine and marital change. When we first spoke, they noted that while they have what might appear to be a traditional division of labor, with Alberto working outside the home and Vero caring for it, they valued communicative joint decision making, which they viewed as progressive. Noting that she "wanted something different" from the life of her ever-pregnant mother and alcoholic father, Vero explained, "To maintain dialogue, we note that we're equal, and that resolves a lot." They had achieved this ability through deliberate, long-term efforts at what they called *desarollo personal* (personal development), a genre of activity that in the United States would be labeled "self-help." This kind of deliberate work on the self has become a hallmark of middle-class efforts to live out modernity worldwide (see, e.g., Freeman 2014).

When discussing Alberto's change over time, both partners told a cohesive story that appeared to be the outcome of their joint work to achieve specific goals for their marriage and their behavior within it. Both said that Alberto was once macho. They attributed this to his upbringing, which the couple had together worked to shed:

VERO: His brothers are machistas.
ALBERTO: Yes, and my father. And I was, too.
VERO: He changed.
EMILY: How?
ALBERTO: We went to therapy three times.
VERO: Yes, he had macho ideas. He would ask, 'What are you spending on this, that?' He wanted to control me, control the spending. He wanted to decide everything. I said that was bad. He didn't hear me. He had to hear it from a third party. So when the psychologist said it, he listened.

Both said this change was fundamental to the current happiness in their marriage, as well as their individual well-being. Alberto noted that he "felt calmer, better" after learning to reject machismo. Their work with a psychologist, along with therapy in Catholic marriage groups that promoted companionate marriage and Vero's ongoing participation in a women's personal development group, enabled them to perform gender in ways that facilitated the progressive and companionate relationship that Vero had always wanted and Alberto had also come to desire.

Further, their collaboration on revising their marital practices in therapy seemed to have set a pattern for shared activity in other life arenas, including health maintenance and medical research participation. In our second interview, they discussed combining exercise with efforts to spend leisure time together, often walking and dancing as a couple. In all of these pursuits, they discussed making continual use of the techniques for avoiding an unequal marital relationship that they had learned in their personal development work. Vero said that their main goal was "to maintain dialogue," because through open communication "we see that we're equal, and that resolves a lot."

When Alberto's work colleagues invited him to participate in the HIM study, they expected that he would be interested because they knew he had personally adopted—and promoted to others—egalitarian, companionate masculinity. He enthusiastically agreed, saying that he had wanted to know his HPV status "for my wife." Further, he encouraged other friends to join, drawing on the idea of couples' biology as he told them that men's testing was important for both partners' health. He also viewed HIM participation as a way to demonstrate difference from his prior machismo and mitigate its health consequences. Regarding learning one's HPV status, he said, "It's machos who don't want to know. Being macho is bad for your health." Alberto's HIM participation was thus a way to highlight and continue living out the companionate responsibility and marriage he and Vero had worked so deliberately to craft.

QUITTING DRINKING AS QUITTING MACHISMO

The majority of the participants and their partners who discussed men's changing performance of masculinity over time identified quitting drinking as a key marker of this shift. This was the case for Rafael, the dental technician, and his office administrator wife, Gabriela. The couple reported a series of family difficulties as they combined their children from previous relationships into one household. They recounted that Rafael's drinking had increased during this tense time, reminding Gabriela of her alcoholic father. "I asked him to change" for the interrelated health of their family and his body, she said. She also framed her request that he stop drinking as a sign of companionate intimacy, "because it shows that I love him, and I care." She wanted Rafael to act more supportively in the home as a parent and spouse and was also afraid "for his health," since he had been diagnosed with precancerous dysplasia in his esophagus.

Rafael's response was to reflect on his own difficult childhood with a heavy-drinking mother and to realize that change was necessary. "[The] changes are for my health," he explained, "but you also have to think of your children. You don't want your kids to suffer what you did. I only went to preparatory school. I'm a medical tech, but I know enough not to hurt my kids. I don't want to teach my daughters to accept bad treatment." Rafael thus framed his shift away from the heavy drinking and emotional withdrawal associated with machismo as a change that conferred modern and high-class status, despite his humble economic and educational background. He further asserted that this change enabled him to better care for his children by modeling companionate responsibility as the attitude they should expect from a husband and father.

Such participants' narratives often reified ideas of the long-suffering woman acting as domestic pillar while men slowly matured. This was the case for the IMSS warehouse worker Reynaldo. "I used to be an alcoholic, and my life has changed a lot," he said. "My wife put up with so much. Thank God I have her. She would have been right to kick me out, but she didn't." He said that he had completely changed after eventually quitting drinking at his wife's request, almost fifteen years earlier. He explained, "There's Reynaldo before and Reynaldo after." While the drinking Reynaldo had lost jobs and failed to support the family economically or to be there emotionally, "Reynaldo after," he said, was a good listener who provided financially and also had positive, intimate familial relationships. He believed he had also successfully modeled this more modern form of masculinity for his sons, albeit by providing a counterexample in their early lives. He joked, "Now my grown sons say they don't want to do the stupid things that I did." Looking back, he noted that "it was my error not to be like that [demonstrating companionate responsibility] from the start, but it's never too late." His wife, a homemaker, emphatically agreed. They saw the HIM study as one of many ways that Reynaldo now contributed to society and showed the kind of helpful, considerate man he had become.

For Alfonso and Elisa, HIM participation was not a reflection of change but a catalyst for it. He worked in construction while she cared for her ailing mother and the couple's home and children while selling shoes from a catalog. They recounted beginning their relationship with what would locally be considered a traditional form of marriage. Alfonso had dated multiple women before deciding he wanted to marry. In contrast, Elisa's strict parents had not allowed her to date. In our first interview, she recalled, "My mother raised us in a way that we couldn't even go out to the corner, or even show our faces out the door." Further, her father was a feared local political leader. "He had a machete, a long one, and a gun, so because of that the boys didn't get close," she recalled. Alfonso was the first man to show romantic interest in her, after meeting her while making a purchase at her family's in-home store. She said, "He came and stayed to talk with me, and that's how it started." While she was not interested at first, she eventually agreed to marry him, because "at the start we got along well." She continued, "One weekend, he came with his parents to ask for my hand. I didn't even know they were coming, but they came, and that was it." Pausing and letting out a rueful and only partially ironic laugh, she concluded, "That was the sad story."

Alfonso's response to my question about how they had decided to marry was quite different. He explained that he had wanted to marry for help with the domestic tasks that he expected a wife to do, from chores to providing company. He said, "I lived alone. For me, it was frustrating to return to an apartment, not have anyone to talk to, to be alone all the time. If I wanted to eat, I had to go to the street or cook myself. Do my own ironing and laundry. So I lacked company more than anything." Thus, both entered into the marriage expecting to conform to traditional gender roles in terms of their tasks and duties, but also hoping that they could find emotional fulfillment. At the point of our first interview, they had been married for twenty years and had three daughters, age eighteen, thirteen, and seven; Elisa's sick mother also lived in their home. Their relationship was distant and rocky.

The lack of emotional closeness appeared to relate to their emphasis on separate spheres of labor. Both agreed that caring for their family through his economic provision and her domestic labor was their most important life task, although they each found their work exhausting. Elisa emphasized the emotional pain of isolation in the home, while Alfonso discussed the physically taxing nature of his job. He said that his family noticed that he got home tired from his physically demanding work and would offer him vitamins. He took them, he said, to "go on" with his work and preserve his health. "More than anything, [I took them] for my daughters," he said. "If I get sick, what will happen to them? Because they're still studying. So I say, 'If I get sick, if something happens to me, what will happen to them? I'm not done caring for them.'" Both saw their own bodies and needs through the lens of their primary duty to care for their family. Meeting those obligations left little time for them to interact. She said, "He leaves for work early in the morning and gets back late in the afternoon, almost at night." He added that brief phone check-ins were their main form of interaction. When I asked in that first interview what they did to have fun together, they sat quietly until she bleakly answered, "Nothing."

Their relationship was also under strain at that time because of their HPV experiences. Alfonso had joined the HIM study because he got genital warts. A doctor told him they were caused by HPV and suggested that he join the study as a means of accessing treatment. When he discussed the experience, he first focused on the "easy" physical aspects, saying, "They just gave me a medicine that I had to put on to burn [the warts] off." He initially glossed over the interpersonal strife his diagnosis had caused, saying that he and Elisa had simply "tried to accept" these new findings and "adapt," because "we've learned how to get over things, over so many years of marriage. How to continue forward through the good and bad."

Yet Elisa challenged this narrative of easy acceptance. Speaking softly and looking only at me, she discussed the emotional toll it had taken on her, especially after she underwent screening that revealed the presence of precancerous cervical lesions and required her to undergo a cone biopsy. She related her anger about the infection to the infidelity that she believed had transmitted it. She said, "It made me really furious, because obviously I was also struck with the infection, contracted because of something that happened outside [of our relationship]." Elisa added that this had taken a toll on their relationship: "I feel like it created some distance between us . . . at least on my part, in terms of us as a couple." After her comments, Alfonso began to discuss the aspects of the experience that had not been as "easy" as his medical treatment. He mentioned his feelings of guilt for cheating and transmitting the virus, saying, "When they did the pap and it came out bad, my conscience really bothered me, you know? Because it was my fault that she was in that situation. I had to explain the cause—that it was because of my error." He also acknowledged Elisa's emotional pain, saying, "She got angry because I was looking in the street for what I had at home."

Over the next year, the couple incorporated such admissions of feelings of anger and guilt into a transformed kind of marital interaction centered on his abandonment of the macho behavior of drinking and partying with his male friends. While their life became more difficult in many ways—Elisa's mother increasingly needed physical care, the construction and sales industries experienced a downturn, and Elisa developed cysts in her breasts—their marriage became notably happier. This was immediately evident in their physical interactions during our second interview. At the first interview, each had sat rigid. In the second, Alfonso often reached out to touch Elisa, tenderly brushing a bug off her arm or a smudge from her chin. This reflected a deliberate shift to more companionate emotional interaction that they reported cultivating through behavioral change. He said that he had dramatically changed his lifestyle: "Now I don't go out alone. . . . If I'm going to have fun, I go with her. Before it wasn't like that. It was me— me here, me there—and now it's not. I go out with her. We go for coffee, go here and there. . . . In our daily life, we've gotten closer." She agreed, adding, "Before, he would go out, not come back, and now, like he says, we go out together. We go for a coffee, end up having a beer or a *Cuba* [mixed drink], end up getting home at ten, eleven at night, one in the morning!" She joked about how they spent so much time together she was always answering his phone: "Now I'm practically his secretary." She also said that they had found new ways to develop their individual interests through this newfound togetherness. Elisa loved to dance, but Alfonso had "two left feet." Now they would go dancing with friends together. He would enjoy chatting while she danced with others, "and he doesn't get mad. Even if he doesn't like to, I can dance."

This emphasis on companionate socialization and the marital happiness it caused continued, even as their economic and family health situations worsened. When we spoke the following year, Elisa recalled an earlier time when she had fantasized about divorce but felt trapped because she could not support their daughters financially. She discussed a radical change since then: "We have united more [since] he changed." The husband who previously "just came home, showered, and left for the street and didn't return until the next day—and drunk, without money," she said, was now even beginning to share the domestic labor. Elisa felt more empowered to ask things of Alfonso beyond economic provision: "One day I said to him, I don't know if you're going to cook or buy something or take us out, but on Sunday it's your turn to take care of the food. So I leave Sundays to him." Looking back, Alfonso located the roots of the shift in his HPV diagnosis and guilt over his wife's cervical cancer scare: "You feel like, swallow me up, Earth! I didn't want to touch her or see her, because you feel guilty." Yet with time "that changed, with increasing closeness between us, because I stopped going around in the street and retired some from alcohol. We started to go out more as a couple, and now if we go out, we go together." Emphasizing that their relationship had moved from a focus on gendered division of labor to communication and intimacy, Alfonso remarked that our interviews had been like "couples therapy, where you come and express what had been done or said between she and I." He added, "It helped me to talk."

Research Participation as a Way for Men to Be Different

In this chapter I have examined the individual level of men's experiences of gendered selfhood, as performed through their involvement in medical research and beyond. Men's narratives about the HIM study's role in their understandings and practices of their own masculinities show that such individual practices of gender are inherently relational. They also reveal which relationships—to which people and groups—men saw as creating, affecting, and being affected by their ways of being men. Male HIM participants overwhelmingly characterized their individual experiences of HPV testing as influenced by and influencing key people in their lives, particularly their wives. Yet their relationships to the imagined, abstract group of "Mexican men" to which they belonged were equally consequential. They generally understood membership in this group as imbuing them with innate tendencies toward machismo. This understanding reified the racialized concept of machismo itself by framing it as natural, if behaviorally modifiable, rather than as an outmoded cultural attitude that could simply be dropped. In keeping with this ideology, they incorporated medical research experiences such as HPV testing into broader efforts to identify and overcome macho tendencies through self-consciously modern practices of masculinity.

By engaging in STI surveillance that framed their bodies as potentially vulnerable, participants reframed intimate testing that they believed more "traditional" men would reject as emasculating into a demonstration of the care for self and others that is central to companionate responsibility. Overall, male participants lived out different takes on the broadly shared pattern of declaring oneself modern by rejecting traits that they associated with traditional machismo. In collaboration with their spouses, men often incorporated medical research experiences into varied daily life efforts to define their own masculinities as "different" from abstract Mexican men's. These assertions of difference signaled, sometimes explicitly and sometimes implicitly, that they had attained more educated, "open-minded," higher-class, and implicitly whiter mestizo status than men who failed to reject inherent urges to machismo. This was true even for men who said they were macho in some ways, such as Javier, who rejected anal sampling but nevertheless claimed status as modern men through their embrace of medical research participation and health care.

Participants also reported relating to the notion of machismo differently over their life courses, with some even radically changing their ways of being men during the HIM study. Some men had always seen themselves as progressive, seeking out partners and forming families that espoused gender equity and companionate relationships. For them, HIM participation was one of many, fairly unremarkable ways to live out and model companionate responsibility. Other men held what they viewed as progressive ideals but sometimes wavered. They understood HPV surveillance as not just a way to show they were modern men, but also as an aid for continuing to be so by making the consequences of being tempted to macho infidelity clear and immediate. Another group of men discussed major changes in their ways of being men over time, as they shifted from performing machismo to companionate responsibility. Giving up drinking and carousing outside their marriages were often hallmarks of this change. Some enrolled in the HIM study after they had changed, in keeping with their new attitudes about masculinity and care. For a few, the HIM study itself served as a catalyst. This was the case for Alfonso, who was prompted to engage in companionate responsibility by his guilt and his wife's anger over her HPV infection following his infidelity.

Participants were also involved in varied patterns of generational change in masculine norms. Some, such as Mario, had spent their lives living out the anti-macho gender ideologies taught by their parents. As I discuss further in chapter 4, Mario and his wife, Paty, deliberately sought to model this attitude for their sons, including through Mario's HIM participation. Conversely, Alberto and Vero had worked collaboratively to craft a companionate marriage, a project that centered on helping Alberto to reject the machismo of his father and brothers and embrace companionate responsibility. After doing much personal development work to accomplish this change over time, Alberto accepted HIM participation as a matter of course.

All of these individual performances of masculinity rested on people's vision of men as part of broader biosocial wholes. Their frequent discussion of machismo indexed a broader and generally implicit racial ideology, described in chapter 1. This is the widely promoted cultural notion that Mexicanness confers innate gendered temperaments and urges that are artifacts of past colonial and Indigenous contributions to an emerging mestizo social body and that, as such, pose barriers to modernization toward an ideally mestizo future on the population level. Participants' discussions of the relationship of their own actions to abstract Mexican machismo thus situated them within a broader Mexican social body and on its leading edge.

Thus, their explicit statements about machismo show how they crafted their own forms of masculinity in implicit reference to beliefs about the influence of Mexican mestizaje on individual biology and temperament, understanding their actions and attitudes as fundamentally shaped by, albeit often through oppositional tension with, the machismo inherent to Mexican men. This finding initiates an analysis that moves outward in levels of scale throughout the rest of this book. Subsequent chapters discuss how men's actions reflected the belief that what they did would directly influence the biosocially interrelated groups to which they belonged. In the next chapter, I discuss how spouses drew on the ideologies of Mexican masculinity discussed here to experience men's HIM participation as direct care for couples, in terms of not only their relationships, but also their ideas of a shared "couples biology" that could be aided by men's STI testing.

THREE

HPV AND COUPLES BIOLOGY

Participants in the Human Papillomavirus in Men (HIM) study and their partners incorporated wide-ranging cultural discourses into their under-standings of human papillomavirus (HPV), from the ideology of machismo discussed in prior chapters to medical explanations provided by HIM study staff. Whenever people learn about a disease, they develop an "explanatory model" for how it works (Kleinman 1980). These models include specific expectations regarding the disease's nature, cause, and course, as well as how and whether it can be treated. These explanatory models reflect not only medical information, but also the other cultural systems of knowledge in which people are immersed, from religion to law and popular culture. For instance, in Mexico, patients' relationships to changing gender ideals often figure into their explanatory models for diverse health conditions (Finkler 1994; Hunt 1998; Yarris and Ponting 2019). Overall, people's explanatory models reflect their internalized cultural expectations and health education; they also change along with new societal developments.

This means that people's understandings of sexually transmitted infections (STIs) are profoundly influenced not just by the medical information they receive, but also by their other ways of thinking about sex and health, including their beliefs about race, gender, and morality. Further, these models are not simply different ways of describing a single, unchanging disease entity. Instead, people construct explanatory models in response to diverse and unique health experiences, and their models, in turn, shape their social and physical experiences of sickness as they suggest specific medical, emotional, and interpersonal responses to new knowledge and bodily experience. Investigating how people create new explanatory models when faced with unfamiliar infections can reveal both how they make sense of new health experiences in light of their existing beliefs and how this process reciprocally influences their emotional and medical responses to STI testing and diagnosis. In this chapter, I argue that HIM participants' and their partners' ideas about how HPV functions reflected and furthered local cultural notions about the embodied consequences of specific kinds of gender and marriage, which, in turn, drew on the racial ideologies underpinning the simultaneous critique and naturalization of machismo.

People's explanatory models of HPV are especially revelatory of these intersections because of the virus's biology and the recent history of HPV-related knowledge and health practice. Later I discuss how several features of HPV-related knowledge in Cuernavaca influenced people's construction of explanatory models of HPV transmission and disease. They include the newness of scientific knowledge about and medical responses to HPV-related cancer; the fact that different HPV strains can have varying health consequences; the unpredictability of whether and when a specific person's infection will cause symptoms; and the focus on women in local HPV-related public health efforts, despite men's and women's equal susceptibility to infection.

The HIM participants' understandings of HPV are also influenced by the fact that STI testing and diagnosis can have major consequences within companionate marriages. For marriages built on ideals of fidelity and openness, unexpected STI findings can disrupt emotional intimacy and raise fears of infidelity. This experience can also threaten the gender performances that companionate marriage requires. In general, sexual health practices can be key ways to assert that one is a particular kind of person (cf. Venables and Stadler 2012), and sexual health problems can compromise efforts to live out desired forms of femininity and masculinity, since they are often linked with impurity, moral failure, and transgression (Hammar 2010). An HPV diagnosis has been shown to generate social stigma and suffering even for asymptomatic patients (Mortensen and Larsen 2010; Waller et al. 2007). Even STI testing without a positive diagnosis has been shown to undermine people's ability to claim desired social identities (Pirotta et al. 2009; de Wit and Adam 2008)—for example, when men's attempts to perform rugged virility are undermined by the implication that their bodies are vulnerable to disease (Shoveller et al. 2010).

Anthropologists have found that people worldwide often base decisions regarding STI testing and disclosure on the impact of these "social risks," rather than on the health or "viral risks" of untreated infection (Hammar 2007; Hirsch et al. 2007: 986; Parikh 2007). However, in some cases STI testing and diagnosis can offer new and positive social possibilities. People can work out ways to reconcile such stigmas with their claims to moral and respectable identities (Gregg 2003). Those with the social status to do so can reject stigmas associated with STI testing, instead using it to demonstrate that they are modern, responsible romantic partners and citizens (Adkins 2001; Biehl et al. 2001; Charles 2013).

This means that STI testing, diagnosis, and disclosure of one's test results to others convey important biological information and also present social risks and opportunities based in broader cultural ideals and stigmas. In Mexico, a powerful history of stigma around STIs coexists with government campaigns that emphasize the moral virtue of testing and education. For example, sexually transmitted infection is often interpreted as a sign of infidelity, meaning that positive diagnosis can threaten both people's attempts to live out companionate marriage and can even destabilize "traditional" marriages, in which infidelity is expected from men but ideally is concealed (Chavez et al. 2001). Conversely, people can attempt to incorporate STI testing and treatment into demonstrations that they are responsible and progressive partners, just as they sometimes use vasectomy or other sexual health practices seen as antitraditional to live out self-consciously modern, companionate marriage (Carillo 2007; Gutmann 2007; Hirsch and Nathanson 2001; see also Pomales 2013). Such efforts at embracing self-consciously modern forms of love and intimacy are ways to assert middle-class or upwardly mobile status amid precarity worldwide (see, e.g., Freeman 2014; Parikh 2016; Tran 2018). Thus, people's explanatory models for HPV reflect their own, context-specific takes on both the social and biological risks and benefits that they understand testing, diagnosis, and treatment to pose.

Here I investigate how HIM participants and their partners developed explanatory models of HPV in response to their preexisting ideas about gender, marriage, and Mexicanness, as well as to the medical information they received. I discuss how their HPV explanatory models linked medical knowledge about the nature of the virus to implicit beliefs about the forms of gender innate to Mexican bodies and their explicit relationships to recent societal critique of the tropes of men as machos and women as long-suffering victims. People's explanatory models for HPV transmission also depended on the happiness of their marriages, especially male partners' ability to live up to the emergent ideal of faithful, companionate responsibility.

Further, their explanatory models drew on a local cultural understanding of individuals as parts of broader collective biologies that they could affect positively or negatively through their own behavior. This included the Mexican social body they believed to be interrelated through a shared racial heritage. It also included what I call "couples biology," the idea that romantic partners' social and physical fates are complexly interlinked, with each person's behavior and bodily status having reciprocal health consequences for the other that can be assessed through biological testing. It is common worldwide to view sex and romantic relationships as vectors for infection risk, based on the obvious biological fact that one partner can transmit an STI to another. I argue that HIM participants' and their partners' concept of couples biology is more extensive than this idea of a dyad in which disease can be transmitted. These spouses understood STI risk within the context of a biosocial view of couples' collective physiology, in which viral transmission was mediated not just by the presence of infection but also by a partner's ability to perform desirably modern gender norms and companionate marriage.

Clinical and Cultural Sources of HPV Knowledge

LOCAL KNOWLEDGE

Existing medical knowledge about HPV, filtered through local ideologies and explanations from HIM study staff, informed participants' and their partners' understandings of the virus. However, the newness and paucity of knowledge and discussion about HPV, as well as the unpredictable consequences of infection, left significant room for interpretation as people crafted their explanatory models. The human papillomavirus only recently entered the public imagination as a health concern. Its links with cancer were discovered in the 1990s, leading to the development of vaccines first approved for use in 2006. Thus, HIM participants often had little or no prior knowledge about the virus's biology. The sexually transmitted strains of HPV are together considered the world's most common STI. They can have widely different health consequences. For most people, HPV infection is asymptomatic. While they can transmit the virus to others, they do not even know they have it unless they undergo testing. Yet for about 10 percent of people, HPV causes health consequences (Centers for Disease Control and Prevention 2013). "Low-risk" strains can cause genital warts, and "high-risk" strains can cause cancer. They most commonly cause cervical cancer but can also cause penile, anal, head, and neck cancer. The biological reasons that certain people develop symptoms and others do not are poorly understood, so they can seem random to both patients and clinicians. Thus, participants often described HPV as "mysterious."

The long and unpredictable time lag between infection and symptom emergence seemed especially mysterious to participants. Genital warts usually first occur in the three months after infection, but it can take months or years for precancerous cellular abnormalities to occur and decades for those to become cancer (Centers for Disease Control and Prevention 2013). Adding to the confusion, it is not known whether infections that become undetectable with current testing technology have actually fully cleared or are simply present in levels too low for the testing to register. This means that people who receive negative HPV diagnoses may have future positive diagnoses that reflect possibly new, but possibly preexisting, infections. Further, people expected condoms to prevent HPV, but they do not actually cover all of the skin that can harbor infection. So sexual encounters that people did not consider possible moments of transmission in fact may have been. This means that a virus contracted years earlier might appear during a more recent sexual relationship, even one in which partners use condoms, leading partners to wonder about the date of transmission.

In addition to the confusion these viral traits can cause, people often misunderstood the role biological sex plays in infection, since both local and global public health practices have encouraged people to see HPV as a women's problem (Daley et al. 2016; Morales-Campos et al. 2018). During the time of my research, the HIM study was the lone site in the area testing men and doing education about men's ability to contract HPV. While the virus infects men and women equally, it is more likely to significantly harm women's health, because cervical cancer is more common than the HPV-related cancers that affect men (Gillison et al. 2008). In Cuernavaca, this emphasis on the relationship between HPV and cervical cancer obscured the fact that men could also contract HPV and also develop related cancers. A well-established national cervical cancer screening program has familiarized people with that disease and fed into cultural ideas that men's macho sexuality harms women's health (Wentzell et al. 2016). This program adopted HPV testing as its main screening method in 2008, becoming Mexico's main source of HPV testing and generating confusion about whether HPV is a cause of or simply another name for cervical cancer (León-Maldonado et al. 2016). The Mexican national vaccination program's focus on girls for HPV vaccination has also spread the idea that only women get the virus and reinforced cultural ideas that women are more physically and socially vulnerable than men.[1]

HIM STAFF EFFORTS TO EDUCATE

Members of the HIM study staff identified these sources of confusion and misunderstanding to me when we discussed their interactions with participants. Staff explicitly attempted to clarify these issues when they explained HPV's biology and health consequences. As clinicians and medical research professionals, they discussed feeling obligated to educate the public about HPV. They also wanted to help HIM participants understand their diagnoses and take appropriate steps to monitor HPV-related health risks. Finally, they hoped to mediate negative social consequences that HPV diagnosis might cause, including emotional and relationship problems and the desire to withdraw from the HIM study.

Staff members sought to destigmatize HPV to spare participants negative emotions and social consequences related to diagnosis. A key way they attempted this was by explaining that HPV was extremely common. The HIM study has found that more than half of Mexican male participants tested positive for some strain of HPV (Giuliano et al. 2008), and staff discussed this and the virus's frequency in the general population to normalize infection. They used metaphors to explain HPV that compared it to other common,

1 Both men and women receive immunity from vaccination against HPV. Yet in Mexico and many other countries, vaccination programs focus on girls as a cost-saving measure based on the (heteronormative) assumption that protecting women from infection will also spare the men with whom they have sex. Unlike in countries where HPV vaccination has generated parental fears regarding promiscuity (Casper and Carpenter 2009) or activated mistrust toward colonial enterprises with histories of threatening local bodies and health systems (Charles 2018; Towghi 2013), in the Mexican context, where people generally view vaccination as a way to access their threatened but constitutionally mandated right to health (Torres-Poveda et al. 2011), the HPV vaccine has been uncontroversial.

natural, and nonthreatening objects. For instance, once of the two study physicians, Dr. Maldonado, often compared the different HPV strains to the branches of a tree.

In response to participants' concerns about the incurability of HPV and the seeming randomness of who would experience symptoms, staff focused on their ability to address symptoms if they arose. The other HIM physician, Dr. Sánchez, said he explained to patients that "there's not an effective way to treat HPV, but we're keeping watch, and the doctor will treat you if there's any change—not to cure the infection, but to treat the change." Similarly, the study manager Jesús reported stressing the "long window that [HPV] has" in his explanations. In introductory discussions with participants, he said, "First we explain that once a virus enters our body, it's difficult to get it out. It's going to be there almost forever, for all our lives, whether its high risk or not." In place of clear answers about why some people develop symptoms, he built on early HIM findings that smoking might increase symptom risk to explain that "everything depends on the quality of life that each person has. We always emphasize that if they have a strong or robust immune system, do exercise, and eat well, they can avoid the risks that lead the virus to begin to transform the cells. If there's a tobacco habit, quit it, stop it, because we all know from the start that [smoking] promotes the growth of the virus and the transformations that the virus starts."

Such explanations also justified the design of the HIM study and highlighted the need for people to continue participating. For instance, Jesús said he explained to participants that "the reason why sometimes [the test] is positive and sometimes it's negative depends on what layer [of tissue] the virus is in, in the moment you take the test. . . . That's why the study is designed this way [longitudinally], so we can make sure and catch the virus when it is [present on the skin]." Jesús told me that, despite these explanations, some participants felt that there was no reason to return to the study after a positive HPV diagnosis since there was no cure and since many believed that only women could be harmed by HPV. Staff members thus stressed the fact that men could get HPV-related warts or cancers and emphasized the need for HPV-positive men to have follow-up visits to address these problems. "We explain to them that at any moment the virus can begin to transform the tissue," Jesús said, "and we emphasize the importance of stopping it in time, because it isn't the same to take off a fragment as to take off the whole penis, for example, or make a bigger hole in the anus or remove the testicles."

The staff broached these worst-case scenarios to increase compliance with return visits, to ensure that men had adequate medical follow-up, and to counter what they saw as the common misunderstanding that HPV could harm only women.

After receiving these explanations, participants and their partners understood the basic medical facts about HPV that HIM staff presented. However, in our discussions they often evinced some confusion about the specifics, especially regarding the nature of HPV types and their relationships to specific disease risks. Participants echoed the staff by characterizing HPV as an STI that could cause cancer; many noted that these were the only aspects of the virus they had heard about before. However, some participants misunderstood the relationship between HPV infection and cancer, seeing HPV as a cancer in itself. For instance, the wholesale worker José understood the virus as an STI but also said, "One supposes that [HPV is] a cancer, right? Human papilloma cancer." Despite these instances of confusion, people usually understood that there were different viral strains with different possible health consequences. Yet while many articulated the concept of different HPV genotypes, others revealed confusion about the relationships among the "different numbers" of HPV types and their possible health consequences. For example, several participants thought that the strain numbers they were given represented the degree to which the virus was present in their body or the relative strength of the virus in their system. Raúl, the lab technician who discusses his acceptance of genital testing in chapter 2, said, "They gave me—there are numbers, right? It was a number that wasn't so bad, you could say not so dangerous. It was a level in an acceptable range, you could say."

Also echoing staff explanations, participants and their partners often discussed the possible asymptomaticness of HPV or the long lag between infection and symptom emergence that HPV infection could have. They frequently used the language of "hiding" or "sleeping" to discuss the virus's latency. In a typical statement, the driver Javier said, "They told me that this problem can be asleep and wake up at any moment." Many also received the message that there could be a long interval between HPV transmission and detection. Raúl's wife, Yolanda, recalled, "They told me that in your first time having sex, you could have contracted it, but the virus doesn't appear until later. Down the road. And because it appeared later, you think you just got it. But that's a lie, because you've had it for some time." As I discuss later, this lag time nevertheless proved socially problematic for many participants.

Both participants' occasional confusion and the lacunae in medical knowledge about who might experience symptoms after how long a time lag left explanatory gaps to fill. Lay and scientific explanatory models always reflect their cultural circumstances. This was especially evident in people's explanatory models of HPV, since they filled these gaps with their preexisting understandings of differences in male and female biology, which, in turn, reflected local cultural assumptions about the gender attributes to which Mexican men and women were innately predisposed. Thus, HIM participants and their partners crafted their explanatory models of HPV from discourses that included HIM staff members' explanations and ideas about health, gender, and sexuality circulating in Cuernavaca. These explanations reflected people's cultural beliefs regarding ideal gender, marriage, and Mexicanness. They also moved beyond clinical accounts of individual bodies being related through sex as a site of infection transmission to cast couples' bodies as single biological units of analysis.

Explanatory Models

SEX-SPECIFIC UNDERSTANDINGS OF HPV BIOLOGY

Participants and their partners incorporated cultural ideas about HPV biology and the nature of Mexican masculinity into their explanatory models of the virus. Since they were involved in a men's HPV study, they did not subscribe to the common notion that only women could get HPV. They nevertheless often believed that women were the ones really harmed by HPV infection. This notion reflected the cultural idea that mestizo biology itself, stemming from racial mixing spawned by conquistadors' rape of Indigenous women, predisposed Mexican men to be machos who would reproduce this history of gendered harm (Gutmann 1996). Men's accounts of efforts to identify and reject innately macho attitudes (see chapter 2) demonstrate the ubiquity and power of this ideology, even among those who consistently live out progressive masculinities in their daily lives. Thus, HIM participants who saw Mexican men as a group as predisposed to machismo extended this ideology to their understanding of HPV biology. Participants commonly viewed HPV-positive men as asymptomatic carriers who could transmit the virus but not be harmed by it and saw women as receptive victims of HPV who were put at risk for cancer. This view was in some ways reinforced by the existence of the HIM study itself. All other local sites for HPV testing and treatment focused on women as possible or current cancer patients, while HIM as the only site for men's HPV testing focused on testing for the virus as an end in itself and included questionnaires that cast men as active agents in viral acquisition and transmission by collecting data primarily about their sexual and lifestyle behavior.

In keeping with the view of men as the active transmitters of HPV, participants and staff members reported that men often joined the study to care for their wives' health. The study manager noted that men enrolled "more than anything else for their partner . . . and their fear that if they have another partner, they can infect them, too." They saw men's testing as care for wives' bodies because they saw men's test results as indicators of the couples' shared viral status. For example, Reynaldo, who worked in the Instituto Mexicano del Seguro Social (IMSS) warehouse, said that, if he tested negative for HPV, "then as a consequence she'll also be OK, it seems to me, right? That's a really interesting point that helped me become a study subject." Similarly, Luisa, an office worker, saw her support of her husband's testing as a way to "take care of us as a couple" and her encouragement of him to continue in the study as a way for her to "take care of myself." This conception of sexual health as a shared attribute of the collective couples biology meant that both partners' well-being could be monitored through the body of either individual spouse.

The common view that men transmitted the virus but women suffered harm also made testing men seem to make sense. Davíd, the IMSS clerical worker quoted in chapter 2 about his belief that HIM participation demonstrated his "open mind," joined the study after he and his wife attended a talk about it at their workplace. As was the case for many participants, Davíd's wife encouraged him to join the study. He explained that they viewed his participation as health surveillance for *her*. "I think that it's only us [men] that transmit the disease," he said, "so if we have it, surely they [our female partners] do, too. So I think that since they haven't detected it in me, my wife is safe."

Davíd extended the ideal that care for men's bodies could help wives in other medical arenas, as well. For instance, when he and his wife had difficulty conceiving, they decided that he should get his fertility checked first, even though it is customary for women to do so. He said, "I'm Mexican but not macho. I'll go to the doctor first, because I know men often blame women for fertility problems." For Davíd, caring for his wife in this embodied way demonstrated that he was a good, not a "macho," man; he believed that "a real man takes care of himself and cares for his partner." His belief that doing the former accomplished the latter was based on his transitive understanding of the couple's sexual and reproductive health status—that one's status would affect the other's body directly. His statements also revealed an explanatory model that tacitly drew on the cultural notion that "Mexican" men as a group were inherently harmful to women, because they harbored regressive tendencies inherited from both rapist conquistador forefathers and unmodern Indigenous heritage. Men such as Davíd voiced the possibility of such harm from even those men who resisted traditional machismo in favor of more modern masculinities.

While HIM participants and their partners generally saw sexual health status as shared rather than individual, they also naturalized the cultural belief that Mexican men and women were biologically and thus behaviorally different. Their understandings of HPV testing and transmission reflected the belief that women were inherently biologically more vulnerable than men. Thus, they usually believed that women were more harmed by HPV than men, and some were unsure whether the virus could harm men as much or at all. Couples often debated this issue in our interviews. This included the taxicab driver Benjamín and nurse Lola, who believed that their desire to engage in health research and education made them different from most Mexicans (see chapter 2). Despite their efforts to engage in positive health behavior, Lola said she thought her husband "had no idea about [HPV] because it only affects the woman." Benjamín responded, "No, the doctor said also [it affects] the man." Lola then presented the common idea that men might have the virus, but women were the ones that it harmed. She argued, "Well, yes, but I'm referring to who it affects, that men are those who transmit it to the woman. The woman, in the end, is at a higher risk for uterine cancer."

Whether or not people believed that HPV could harm men, there was consensus that the virus harmed women more. This is accurate in the sense that HPV-related cancers are more common in women than men, yet participants often based this belief not on cancer prevalence data but on the understanding that women's bodies were inherently more vulnerable to disease than men's. For instance, Raúl saw his genital warts as "no big deal" for his own health, but he advocated for health monitoring for his wife because he believed that the HPV strain he had "can advance further in women." Similarly, Yolanda's husband's positive diagnosis made her "a little bit afraid" because, she said, "My husband explained that it's worse in women. It's more, it can do more harm than in men." Some participants extrapolated these ideas into their understandings of HPV vaccine performance, with several believing, as a lawyer noted, that the vaccine "in the case of men is curative" rather than simply preventative. This notion of sex-specific vaccine function reflects a belief that HPV was simply less significant and harmful to men's bodies.

This belief was reinforced by the HIM staff's recommendation that men diagnosed with high-risk HPV strains urge their wives to enter cervical cancer screening, while screening programs did not exist for the cancers that men might face. Couples thus experienced men's diagnoses as the start of women's long-term medical scrutiny. Describing a typical outcome of a man's positive test result, Eusebio, an electrician, recounted, "The doctor said that I needed to talk with my wife and inform her that I'd gotten a positive in the study and as a consequence of that, well, she'd have to be under constant surveillance."

The participants and partners who did come to see HPV as risky for men as well as women reported finding that information surprising. For instance, Reynaldo said that the idea that HPV posed a disease risk to men "was something new; we as men think that it's something specific to women." He remembered his "surprise" at learning from a study recruitment talk that although "normally you think that this virus only affects women . . . men can also be affected. That's why they're doing this study." Even men who discussed male HPV risk continued to foreground the risk for women, as when an IMSS lab technician said that the study was useful because "it's important to know if you're a carrier, since you can give it to the woman and also get cancer." Thus, while a few participants incorporated the idea that HPV can harm men into their explanatory models, even their explanations reflected the widespread assumption that men are simply, biologically, harmful to women, who are innately vulnerable.

MEN AS CARRIERS

The HIM staff expressed frustration that, despite their emphasis on men's risk of genital warts and cancer, participants and their partners tended to focus solely on cervical cancer. They also sought to disrupt the common narrative that men were asymptomatic HPV carriers and women potential cancer victims. They often explicitly cast HPV transmission and disease risk as sex-neutral. For example, Jesús, the study manager, often described transmission as "a mutual responsibility." Nevertheless, he said:

> Women put the guilt on the men, Because men are more promiscuous—because of that, right?—even when they do the questionnaire and [the women] also have multiple partners. . . . What happens at the root of this is that before [medicine] didn't have a real understanding of what the virus can cause in the man. Now we know that the virus affects both equally. . . . That breaks the paradigm and takes [the participants] work

to understand. And even after the explanation and when we tell them and sometimes spend up to two hours with one, they can't get that idea out of their head.

Jesús's comment reveals how cultural expectations of Mexican men, as biologically predisposed by their mestizo natures to be macho and "more promiscuous" than women, were naturalized even in the comments of a staff member explicitly critiquing sex-specific ideas of HPV risk.

Similarly, Dr. Maldonado noted, "Generally, the woman blames the man." She thought this was a consequence of "disinformation and bad information. We try to convince them otherwise, but they don't hear us." However, she also saw a change in people's ideas over time. Previously, there were "many myths" about HPV, including that only men could transmit it and that men were born with HPV that they passed on to women, she said. Further, women used to think, "I'm the victim, I don't transmit." By 2015, after several years of the HIM study and school-based HPV vaccination, Dr. Maldonado said, "people know more." Yet just a year earlier, in the final full round of participant interviews, people continued to reproduce the narrative of sex-specific transmission that she critiqued. For instance, the factory manager Adalberto explained, "It's always the woman who has the problem. . . . [W]hen that happens to her is always when they detect [HPV] in the man. Now we see that we are, like, the provider [of the infection]." Here he fuses expectations of men as sexually harmful and as active economic providers, framing them as providers of a dangerous virus.

Thus, despite explanations by HIM staff, participants generally saw men as carriers and women as symptomatic victims of HPV. Couples often reported that a man's positive diagnosis was primarily significant in terms of the danger it might signal for his female partner. Some participants even incorporated this idea into their understanding of the logic of the HIM study, as when Adalberto said that he thought the study focused on men "because I think that it's only us who transmit this disease."

Participants' language usage reflected their gendered understandings of the different effects HPV could have on male and female bodies. This was especially linguistically visible since in Spanish the word for "carrier" has masculine and feminine forms. Seven people—five men and two women—used the term *portador* (male carrier). Almost all of them used this term in their initial interviews, when they discussed the broad contours of their emotional and interpersonal experiences relating to HPV. People tended to use the term as they discussed the negative aspects of masculinity and male biology that they believed made men the likely carriers of the virus.

Some men voiced gendered guilt about being a portador that was linked to ideas of male biology as harboring and transmitting asymptomatic HPV. For example, Lino, a factory worker, explained when we met: "I'm the carrier, the problem that causes the virus, for all the deaths there have been and why my wife is in this position." When I responded that it sounded like he felt guilty, he said he did, because even though he did not infect his wife intentionally, "It's my fault, right?" He added that the man "is the one that carries, and you [the woman] only get hurt. [The man] is the one that transmits, it's easy because nothing happens to me. I go on infecting." In this case, it did appear that Lino had been the first to contract HPV, since he had had other sexual partners during breaks in his early relationship with his wife, while she had slept only with him (although the fact that nonpenetrative genital contact can spread HPV makes it difficult to definitively identify transmission histories). However, the shifts in Lino's language between discussion of himself and a universal man who "carries" and "goes on infecting" suggest that his guilt relates more to his general idea of men's behavioral and biological natures than to his specific sexual history. His characterization of men as unfeeling infectors mirrors local critiques of macho Mexican men as heartless serial womanizers.

While the IMSS clerical worker Francisco did not feel personal guilt for transmitting HPV (and, as discussed in chapter 2, used his recent negative test results to recommit to fidelity), he nevertheless spoke about perceived differences in the course of the virus in male and female bodies in a language of gendered blame. He said that he entered the study "principally for [my wife]," and that both of them hoped to learn "whether or not I was a carrier of the virus." They believed his testing was important because "the man is the carrier and the woman is the one who pays, right? The one who has the consequences." Similarly, the IMSS lab technician José Luis said that he learned from a HIM study recruitment talk about HPV and STIs that, as men, "we're carriers of viruses, so we have to be checked." He became especially concerned when he learned that the genital wart he had had removed thirty years earlier could be a sign of a permanent infection and thus felt guilt and "anguish" when he discovered that he was a portador.

Other men discussed fears that being a carrier made them dangerous to women in ways that they associated with problematic machismo. They often discussed viral transmission in the same terms they would a deliberate act of gendered harm, such as domestic violence. Further, their statements suggested that embodying this kind of damaging masculinity made them feel worse about themselves as men. Several men talked about the realization that they could cause "danger" to women, as when José Luis also said that being a carrier "is a really worrisome problem; it lowers your self-esteem. You think, am I dangerous?" Similarly, a mechanic said that he sought testing because "I wanted to know if I could harm my partner." In another twist on feelings of failed masculinity, José Luis said that his diagnosis and the wait to see whether his wife would have a bad pap smear result "was impotence, because you can't do anything." Such comments reveal fears that even men striving to be progressive and perform companionate responsibility could be thwarted by the regressive aspects of masculinity they implicitly attributed to mestizo biology through discussions of innate machismo.

To varying degrees, all of these men voiced desires for companionate relationships and framed themselves as caring for their wives, families, and health in ways that challenged stereotypical machismo. Some thus experienced "being a carrier" as an identity rooted in problematic Mexican male nature, which compromised their efforts to be good men by suggesting that they had engaged in negatively macho behaviors. José said that he was both incredulous and disheartened about his positive diagnosis, since he linked HPV positivity to promiscuity:

> I've lived my life trying to abstain from certain things, in my married life. My wife and I try to respect each other, more than anything. Many times, one has the opportunity to have another partner. . . . I always say no. I always try to conserve the respect I have for [my wife]. Even though she's not with me wherever I go, I act as if she were with me, and that makes me feel good. I feel satisfied that I've been able to live well . . . , so in this aspect of contagion and transmission and all that, it made me think that, we'd suppose that this person [meaning himself] is good but inside of myself, I'm not going to feel good.

José was somewhat comforted by a staff member's response to his questions about HPV transmission, reporting, "The doctor said that it's not a sign of living a bad life [*maluso de su vida*], but that it develops in some people, not others."

Overall, fifteen of the twenty couples or individuals interviewed who discussed their explanatory models of HPV transmission believed men to be the sole or main transmitters of the virus or believed that HPV was significantly more harmful to women. Only one couple and one woman interviewed alone used the term *portador* in a gender-neutral or morally neutral way. Guadalupe, a homemaker, understood being a carrier as different from truly having HPV. When I asked whether her husband "had a positive diagnosis," she replied, "Not positive. He's a carrier, but he still doesn't have any symptoms." In a relationship that she characterized as trusting and faithful, she said that this knowledge seemed "normal—you just have to get checked and deal with it." The couple who used the term portador neutrally also discussed the idea that women could be HPV carriers, or portadoras. Javier, the driver, and his partner, Francisca, met after he had joined the study (and after he had overcome the initial discomfort he discusses in chapter 2), so he had explained that experience and discussed HPV early in their relationship. He recalled, "I explained to her that I was participating in a study with the aim of getting to understand this virus, or sickness, to find a possible vaccine. But at that time what I understood was that I might be a carrier, but not active." She then hoped to join the proposed women's HPV study to "learn whether I'm a carrier to get early treatment" if necessary. However, both saw study participation as primarily an altruistic act that supported medical research.

As with Javier and Francisca, the few people who used the word *portadora* framed being a carrier as a possible trait of both women and men. Even though people often discussed women "having" or "being at risk for" HPV, which implied passive exposure to the virus, only three participants used the more active term *portadora*. All were female, and two of the three did not use it until their final interviews. Even women who had been diagnosed with HPV as part of cervical cancer screening before their husbands entered the study tended not to use *portadora*, because characterizing people as carriers generally seemed to connote a deliberate lack of care for one's partner that made cultural sense as a masculine but not as a feminine trait. Overall, it appears that participants generally saw being a carrier as a male attribute, but over time, and after learning about HPV in the course of the study, a very few came to see it as a simple marker of having an inactive virus rather than a condition based in male biology and naturalized ideas of problematic male behavior.

EXCEPTIONS

In contrast to these common beliefs, a few couples did develop explanatory models in which men and women were equally responsible for and vulnerable to harm from HPV transmission, in support of their explicitly stated political commitments to gender equity. This was the case for the researcher Roberto and school administrator Griselda. They told me that they had joined the study to receive HPV testing that they hoped would help them to rebuild trust after her idea of opening their relationship sexually had left them on the brink of separation. While they initially thought that their liberal attitudes would make open marriage possible, they found their relationship challenged by emotional attachments to other partners. They said that the growing mistrust between them was symbolized by the need to use condoms—a literal barrier between them—in case either had contracted an STI. The couple hoped that negative HPV test results (which they could not procure for him anywhere but the HIM study) would enable condomless sex and spark reconciliation. In their understanding, both partners were equally self-determining in their sexual actions, equally capable of STI transmission, and equally vulnerable to both the biological and emotional harms presented by their spouses' extramarital sex.

In this light, Roberto criticized the design of the HIM study for focusing only on men's actions. He noted that the sexual behavior questionnaire "asks how many partners *you* had, but it's not only an issue of one person if your partner isn't trustworthy. There's a question about, did you have sex with someone other than your primary partner and get a disease, but not about if your partner was unfaithful and you got a disease." He extended this critique of the medical study's understanding of sexuality as an individual action rather than a partnered interaction by further noting that it reflected gender stereotypes by casting men as the main actors in the realm of sexuality. He added that since women cheat on men, as well as vice versa, assuming that only men have multiple partners is sexist. Thus, Roberto and Griselda's view that partners shared equal responsibility for sexual activity and other aspects of a relationship was directly reflected in their explanatory model of HPV transmission and potential harm. Both this model and their analysis of the HIM study's design incorporated their shared critique of local cultural assumptions about gender.

Couples' Responses to HPV

AVOIDING BLAME

Participants' explanatory models of HPV biology were not the most significant determinants of how men's diagnoses affected their relationships. Their responses instead mirrored the broader cultural belief that Mexican men were innately predisposed to machismo but could achieve individual and societal growth by resisting that bodily predilection and behaving well. While most people saw men as carriers and women as biological victims of

HPV, whether or not they saw positive diagnosis as problematic for their own relationship depended on men's behavior rather than viral status. Spouses who agreed that men had behaved well, in "modern" and anti-macho ways, resisted assigning moral blame to male partners. This was true even for couples in which one or both partners developed an HPV-related lesion that required medical attention.

Many avoided assigning guilt by framing HPV as a medical condition like any other, avoiding the stigma related to its sexual route of transmission. This was the approach taken by the dental technician Rafael, whose efforts to quit drinking and understanding of STI testing as "embarrassing but necessary" are discussed in chapter 2. When I asked him whether his positive diagnosis and removal of possibly HPV-related lesions had affected his marriage, he said it had not. His wife, Gabriela, an office administrator, added, "No. I feel that [it's like] you have a hernia and you operate. It's a thing that happens, and it depends on how you deal with it." Similarly, some couples described undergoing medical surveillance as a way to keep an HPV diagnosis from affecting their marriage. A systems engineer said that diagnosis "really hasn't affected us, . . . because we've taken it maturely. . . . We've taken it as something natural. We're conscious of it, and we try to take preventative actions." By focusing on mutual support through health problems and on engaging jointly in preventative health care, couples used HPV diagnoses as opportunities for living out progressively modern health behavior and relationships focused on understanding and care. It appeared that while people understood the biological aspects of HPV transmission through their generic ideas of the abstract Mexican man's biological predisposition to harm women, they evaluated issues of intentionality and guilt in viral transmission in light of actual men's gender performances. For HIM participants, these were often efforts at self-consciously nontraditional, companionate marriages.

Many couples explicitly framed their responses to HPV positivity as demonstrations of their marital closeness and as ways for men to perform companionate responsibility. For instance, Pedro, a taxicab driver, said that it "was easy" to tell his wife about his diagnosis, "because she's my partner. I don't have any secrets from her." Couples often discussed deliberately engaging in processes of working through fear or the tendency to blame to support each other in accordance with their vision of how spouses should behave.

This was the case for the IMSS employee Leo, who was quoted in chapter 2 discussing the need to normalize HPV testing, and his wife, Flor. Leo had received a high-risk-positive diagnosis in the HIM study. He described that experience as something he and his wife had to work together to solve, in the same way they collaborated to address other challenges. Extending the language of companionate marriage to the HPV experience, he said, "Here, if we can support each other, that's the best. And I think that would also be true if there was some sickness [caused by HPV]. It wouldn't cause distance between us. You always need to be with the person." Flor discussed the process by which she drew on this philosophy, as well as her experience working as a nurse, to come to terms with the news about the diagnosis. She said, "When he told me, at first I said, 'No!' It scared me. But then I said, 'Well, take it calmly, investigate what's happening.' So I did research, in books and on the internet. And I said, 'OK, this has a solution, and it's better than not knowing.'" She discussed consciously mediating between her thoughts "as a woman," that "I'm going to contract this, I can die," and her understanding as a nurse that "these things have solutions" so "nothing will happen" as long as both she and Leo attended to their health. She reported that ensuring that both of them were "getting the appropriate care"—Leo being continually checked in the HIM study, and Flor getting pap smears to detect precancerous cervical lesions—helped them to deal with the situation calmly. Thus, Flor acknowledged the temptation to adopt a gendered explanatory model that cast Leo as the cause of harm and herself as a victim, but she worked deliberately to reject it in favor of a narrative emphasizing mutual support.

Their joint development of an explanatory model of HPV as a neutral medical issue to be dealt with collaboratively emerged from their use of this approach more broadly in their marriage. Flor noted that her concerns were allayed by the fact that "we have trust, we talk," so they could work through their fears together by drawing on the information about his biological state they received from the HIM study. Leo noted that the fact that there was no change in his condition "calmed me down," as did the fact that his wife was able to "take this calmly." He greatly admired her approach to his positive results, saying, "She has a lot of knowledge," as well as an "other vision" from the average person, regarding their shared health and life in general, and the meaning of HPV specifically. While he had felt guilt for potentially transmitting the virus, "to the point of considering if it would be better for us to separate" to protect her, they were able to talk about their emotions, as well as her research about HPV, to "calm down."

Both said that this experience was typical of their problem-solving strategy as a couple. While they might have transitory fears or concerns, he noted, they sought to "support each other" so they could "always be together." In fact, the following year they reported employing this same strategy to deal with the complicated birth of their second child, who was delivered early, by cesarean section, after Flor developed preeclampsia. Again, they stressed that they had both felt frightened and confused but coped by seeking out health information and discussing it together. Flor said, "You can face things better together. One of you might be worried about something, and the other can calm them down. Instead of arguing, we unite."

Other couples struggled more to reframe HPV diagnoses in ways that enhanced, rather than undermined, their efforts at companionate marriage. Many in this situation experienced a period of emotional difficulty and marital strife but then consciously worked together to face the diagnosis; this shared coping effort itself represented a return to companionate ideals. For instance, before he was diagnosed with HPV, the factory worker Marco mused that having the virus would be difficult because spouses were so intertwined. "Transmitting it to my partner would affect my mood," he said. "It would affect me if she were affected." However, his homemaker wife, Ginebra, said that, because of the shared nature of both the virus and their life together, she would take a positive diagnosis in stride. If he were positive, "obviously I would be, too," she said. "But more than anything I would tell him to buck up, to support him and cheer him up, and if there is a treatment or cure, [I'd say,] 'Well, let's go, not stay here stagnant.'" Two years later, both partners did test positive for HPV, and Ginebra required follow-up care. Contrary to their expectations, this caused strife.

Marco and Ginebra's ire rested on two key points. The first was the idea of spouses' sexual health statuses as inherently interlinked, with one's actions affecting the other. From that perspective, one person contracting HPV was directly harming the shared couples biology. This explains Marco's statement that, upon diagnosis, each initially focused on "finding the guilty party or putting the guilt on one side." The second point is the stigma associated with STIs, including cultural assumptions that STI carriers are morally suspect or, as is a common belief in Mexico, that STI positivity is a sign of infidelity. From this perspective, Marco added that positive diagnosis had been a *golpe moral* (moral blow). Thus, the couple faced a period of interpersonal difficulty when their positive diagnoses seemed to indicate divergence from their companionate ideals of faithful intimacy and the ability to easily talk through emotional difficulties. However, they focused on cultivating the latter ability. Marco said, "We decided that we would face it, and make an effort, that what had happened, and that we were going to be here together and forever." Through this conscious recommitment they deliberately sought to enact the sort of companionate relationship and response to health difficulties that they valued.

Couples in which both partners had had sex with others before they married most explicitly incorporated HPV positivity into self-consciously modern takes on relationships. For instance, Araceli, an accountant, said that while "the surgery was very painful" to remove a papilloma, she was not angry at her husband for transmitting HPV. She noted, "I already knew he'd had three partners [before we married]." However, it is also important to note that couples and individuals sometimes held multiple, competing views about HPV's social meanings simultaneously. While she did not place moral blame on her husband for transmitting HPV, he felt significant guilt. As discussed earlier, Lino, the factory worker, identified himself as "the carrier," which he also understood to make him as a man "the problem" that could harm his wife. Thus, people's statements in interviews about the nature and significance to relationships of HPV transmission reflect particular moments within their ongoing discussions and reconsiderations of the social consequences of HPV.

In a context where the ideal of female virginity upon marriage has only relatively recently been contested (Amuchástegui Herrera 1996), some couples used acceptance of HPV positivity to challenge both ideals of women's purity and the notion that men alone transmit the virus. This was the case for Paty and Mario, introduced in chapter 2. Mario, a bartender, told me that he joined the study in part because his wife, Paty, had previously had an HPV-related lesion removed. They reported configuring both partners' related medical experiences as venues for living out marital intimacy and support. Mario said he went with Paty to gynecological visits: "There have also been occasions when she's going to get her pap smear, when they put in the little camera, and I'm there every time." He then said that Paty had accompanied him to his first HIM visit to provide moral support. Paty concluded, "There aren't many taboos between him and me."

Given this context of mutual support, both said they were uninterested in the question of who had first contracted the virus. "I was never interested in meeting a virgin woman," he said. "I don't see why she has to be a virgin. I don't see the point. It's a membrane. It can break in any moment, without it even being caused by sexual relations." Paty added that, while the diagnosis was stressful due to health concerns, they did not see it as a relationship problem. Mario said, "There weren't reproaches because I'd had partners. She had also sexual partners before we lived together, so why make martyrs of yourselves?" Paty concluded his thought by saying, "Lo que no fue en tu año, que no te haga daño"—literally, "If it didn't happen during your time, it doesn't do you any harm," or, colloquially, "That's ancient history."

Thus, while most participants' explanatory models of HPV transmission reflected the idea that Mexican male biology was inherently harmful to women, their social responses to HPV positivity reflected the notion that progressively modern men would struggle against innate machismo. In cases where men were engaging in faithful, companionate relationships, and thus acting in contrast to the base machismo generally assumed to be biologically innate to Mexican men, partners deliberately strove to understand HPV diagnosis as an opportunity for mutual openness and care rather than gendered blame.

USING COMMUNICATION TO COPE WITH DIAGNOSIS

Examples such as these also demonstrate that couples used interactions regarding men's varied HIM study experiences to live out companionate ideals of communication and openness. Participants frequently discussed the value of talking through problems, including those related to intimate health and sexual issues. Often when I asked couples what they did when times were hard, they responded, "We talk." People frequently used the word "communication" when discussing both the best qualities of their relationship and their experiences dealing with difficulties. This was the case for Luisa, the office worker quoted earlier in the chapter, and her husband, Pedro, an industrial technician. They identified "talking" as their main technique for resolving marital stress and proudly discussed communicating with their friends about Pedro's HIM participation and test results. Luisa said this openness was helpful, because "people are less afraid of things when they ask about them, because it's better to know." Pedro added, "Also, maybe because of our education, we're likely to talk about things." Discussing their health and emotional experiences with friends was thus a way to work through issues while demonstrating their modern and educated communication style.

Of course, claiming to communicate openly can be different from actually doing it. Instead, self-consciously seeing oneself as practicing intimate communication is a way of performing the desirable traits associated with modern marriage and family, which might not actually involve complete openness. For instance, Benjamín shared all of his HIM results with Lola, including his positive HPV diagnosis, and both agreed that open communication had helped them see this as a health issue rather than an interpersonal problem. Both also agreed that Benjamín had become a better partner over the course of their marriage, coming to focus fully on their domestic life and acting as a deeply engaged father. However, Lola believed that prior infidelity had caused Benjamín's HPV infection and that it was his shift to becoming faithful that had led to his improvement as a husband. Despite his frankness about his STI status, Benjamín followed the common cultural script for vehemently denying that he had ever been unfaithful to Lola. Thus, "communication" is more a strategic performance of modernity and intimacy than a practice of complete transparency.

Even so, participants' commonly stated desire for open communication, and their frequent practices of it—including the disclosure of men's test results—demonstrates the importance of this quality to most study participants. Disclosure of potentially stigmatizing information such as STI positivity is not a given in any relationship. It is especially not a given in Mexican cultural contexts, where families often deal with potentially stigmatizing sexual or health information, from children's homosexuality to men's infidelity, by treating it as an open secret that is widely known but never discussed (Carillo 2002; Hirsch et al. 2002). Yet only a very few couples in my study appeared to use the open secret model to keep evidence of men's infidelity from intruding in the lived daily experience of their relationships with each other. Instead, spouses often engaged in disclosure—of not only test results but also interpersonal difficulties and sexual transgressions—as a key practice of companionacy.

The importance of disclosure to their senses of themselves as intimately interconnected is highlighted by moments when a spouse thought the other had failed to be fully open. For example, Pablo, an IMSS physician, said he did not mention his positive HPV test to his wife, Theresa, because "I took it as a false positive—it was only one test out of ten. It wasn't important." Yet Teresa, a homemaker, took it as a serious breach of trust when she saw the test result among his papers. She said she was angry because "he kept his own council. Why didn't he have the trust to tell me?" Because she thought he had tried to hide the result, she worried that he had been unfaithful and saw that as a problematic "lack of trust" within their otherwise happy marriage.

To demonstrate openness, couples in the study went out of their way to discover whether men were HPV-positive and to jointly assess their test results. They did so in part to show that they were different from those couples who kept secrets or conformed to problematically traditional marital practices such as male dominance or the use of open secrets to avoid direct communication. They sometimes highlighted this distinction by contrasting their marriages with those of people who had divorced over HPV. This was the case for Adalberto, the factory manager, who told me, "I have a cousin who had HPV, and it destroyed her marriage. They separated. It was because of her husband: he was living crazily, getting into things he shouldn't have. That affirms my desire not to be with other people. It's an example of what can happen. These things can happen, and they do if you don't take care of yourself." Through this statement, Adalberto asserted his difference from his cousin's macho husband and characterized his own marriage as strong enough to weather HPV testing because he was faithful and he and his wife maintained respect and communication.

ASSIGNING BLAME

Unlike the people who sought to avoid blame to practice the open communication they saw as a hallmark of companionate marriage, women who felt their husbands had failed to conform to modern ideals of marriage and masculinity developed explanatory models that blamed negative male behavior, as well as biology, for HPV transmission. This was especially the case when wives knew or suspected that their husbands had been unfaithful. While the long dormancy period of HPV often made it impossible to know medically which partner had first contracted the virus and when it had happened, couples who had experienced male infidelity often assumed that to be the mode of transmission. Women who believed that their spouses had cheated drew on the cultural tropes of "traditional" Mexican masculinities as harmful to women, along with explanatory models of viral transmission based on those ideas. For example, Ana-María, a hairdresser, said that "the man has to be conscious. If he has [HPV], if he's unfaithful, this is a difficult problem that has consequences, because he can bring the problem to his house and his partner. And the partner has a greater possibility of getting cancer." Turning to the husband she believed was cheating, she said pointedly: "They have to be conscious, if I'm speaking in general terms, because the woman is more affected than the man." Knowing that HPV could be asymptomatic for long periods, Ana-María added, "Even if he was unfaithful twenty years ago, it could be that before, because he was young and in good health, [the virus] wasn't detectable. . . . [Transmitting HPV years later] would be terrible, because, for example, I've been faithful my whole life. And imagining that one would pay the consequences of the youthful actions of one's husband is terrible." Through such thinly veiled hypothetical statements, Ana-María used our interview as a forum for critiquing her husband for the interrelated emotional and physical harm she felt he had caused her by failing to be "conscious" of his actions and capitulating to his base nature.

Using a similar discursive style, the homemaker Elena reminded her husband, Eusebio, that his actions had caused harm that she felt rose to legally actionable levels. As she recapped their difficult thirty-eight-year marriage and his HPV positivity in our final interview, she mused, "If he's a carrier, if he has that, well, I imagine that I do, too. So I thought, 'What if I sue him?'" This notion demonstrates that she held Eusebio accountable for the bad behavior that she felt had put her at risk. He admitted to being unfaithful for much of their marriage, noting in our first interview, "Without a doubt, we've had some friction because of my living freely outside the house. We've had periods of [marital] abstinence because of anger, because of reproaches about 'Where are you going?' and 'Who are you with?'" Elena interjected, "Well, we had abstinence precisely because I was thinking about how he could bring in some health problem from outside, which is what happened to me in the end, right?" She directly cast his negative masculinity as a threat to her health.

Elena's threat of divorce, together with their conversion to evangelical Christianity (discussed at length in chapter 6), eventually led Eusebio to rethink his sexual behavior. Looking back as an older man, he said, "[Over time] I stopped myself from looking for other women." He framed his urge to infidelity as a natural trait that he sought to overcome through willpower and prayer and described his positive HPV test results as an additional aid for sexual continence. He said, "Now, the knowledge that I'm a carrier, it made me think that it isn't fair to trouble another woman and make her run the risk of catching this problem. I did that more than once, and I suppose in some way, I thought, 'I brought this problem into my house, and now I'll leave it there.'" Both spouses thus agreed that men's infidelity and innately problematic masculinity had been the root cause of the introduction of an STI into their home. Of course, this agreement that Eusebio was to blame did not put an end to their strife, because Elena remained unconvinced of his sincere commitment to change. This was demonstrated by her fantasy of suing him for the harm he had caused her, which she broached two years after he had claimed in our interview to have fully changed. Her lingering anger revealed both that emotional hurt could persist despite claims of change and that wives of cheating husbands were often unconvinced that such claims were truthful.

This common association of HPV transmission with men's infidelity also influenced men's fears about their own positive diagnoses. Despite the commonly held belief that HPV posed only a minor biological risk for men, it posed significant social risk specifically because it was associated with bad male behavior in general, and infidelity in particular. For example, Adalberto feared that a current positive diagnosis might result from youthful indiscretion and make it seem as if he had not in fact changed his way of being a man in the ways he now valued. He said that his negative results "made us feel more secure, both for her and myself." This security came not just from knowing that the couple's body was free from viral risk, but also from the elimination of the social risk of HPV positivity. He explained, "Now I'm like one of those old people, [with] my partner only and no one else. But, still, despite that, you have that fear, right? Because you could have been infected, and you don't know when." Even though he said he had been raised to be faithful and now knew that "there is nothing better than respect" shown for one's wife by "not going from bed to bed," Adalberto had nevertheless feared HPV positivity as a consequence of more youthful faltering between "going for the bad or the good" in his sexual behavior. Yet he found HIM participation to be worth the social risk of diagnosis, because, as discussed earlier, he believed that only men transmit HPV and that the virus specifically harms women. "The security [testing] gives you" is worth it, he said, "as much for me as for my wife." Given his negative results, he no longer had to fear being a portador or that his wife would suffer health problems caused by his past bad behavior.

Gendered Ideas of Biology Influence Explanatory Models and Social Risk of HPV

Ideas about HPV's biology and the social consequences of HPV diagnosis among HIM participants and their partners reflect changing and contested ideas about gender and marriage in Cuernavaca. Participants who discussed their explanatory models of HPV tended to understand it as a virus that men transmitted to women, who, in turn, were the major group subject to harm. The fact that cervical cancer is both more common and better known than the HPV-related cancers that harm men and that women's bodies are implicitly framed as more vulnerable than men's in sex-specific HPV vaccination and screening programs contributed to this view. However, those were not the only factors shaping participants' explanatory models. To create explanatory models of HPV, HIM participants and their partners also drew on ideals of companionate marriage, as well as beliefs that men might be predisposed to infidelity and women, to vulnerability. This was evident in the blame- and guilt-ridden language they used to discuss male portadores; their ideas of one-way transmission from men to women; and the persistence of the belief that only women could be harmed by HPV, despite HIM clinicians' efforts to stress that both sexes could transmit and be harmed by the virus. As is the case with men's duties to perform invulnerability in other settings (Reihling 2020), participants' notions of men's invulnerability to HPV relative to women actually made men vulnerable to specific forms of emotional suffering related to the guilt of portador status.

Overall, participants and their partners crafted their explanatory models of HPV from several sources: medical information they had received about the virus, assumptions about HPV gleaned from the woman-focused Mexican vaccination and screening programs, and implicit beliefs about the biologically innate predispositions toward male machismo and female victimization that many sought to reject in their performances of gender and marriage. Beyond simply reflecting these discourses, people's explanatory models influenced their ongoing social and physical experiences of HPV testing and diagnosis by providing frameworks for interpreting and reacting to medical information and bodily change.

People's explanatory models of HPV also fundamentally rested on their notions that spouses were enmeshed in collective couples biologies. In this way, their ideas differed fundamentally from the individually focused explanatory models of the virus that HIM clinicians presented, which reflected biomedicine's focus on the individual body as the site of infection and treatment. Participants' and their partners' understandings of the consequences that one spouse's HPV positivity would have for the other went beyond the notion that sex could transmit the virus between partners. Instead, most conceptualized spouses' bodies as parts of a single biological system, in which one partner's viral status necessarily mirrored the other's, meaning that testing one partner for HPV was the same as testing both.

This notion reflected beliefs about the fundamental interconnectedness of the Mexican social body discussed in the prior chapter, envisioned as an entity composed of individuals sharing a set of biological and social traits and whose embodied fates could be influenced by the others to whom they were linked. It also reflected the idea that emotional interconnectedness and open sharing of thoughts and feelings were fundamental to companionate marriage. Thus, participants who saw themselves as modern Mexicans expected to be interrelated with their partners in both body and mind. In subsequent chapters, I discuss the ways that not only this idea of the couples' body, but also people's conceptions of families and communities as biosocially integrated entities that together compose the Mexican social body as a whole, influenced participants' and their partners' experiences of and hopes for specific benefits from HIM participation. Further, while I focus here on HPV transmission as a key example of a health condition understood to exist at the level of the couple rather than the individual, people also deployed the idea of couples biology to understand other health experiences, such as the struggle with infertility that Davíd discussed.

However, while this notion of couples biology led people to understand HPV positivity as a shared status, they expected the viral and social harm potentially posed by the virus to be unequally shared based on gender. This, too, reflects local cultural understandings of the broader social body. Specifically, it reflects the notion that innately harmful masculine traits inherited by mestizo men from conquistador forefathers—and as members of a group that hoped to modernize away from Indigenous gender norms viewed as backward—pose risk to mestiza women and, as I discuss in later chapters, threaten the advancement and health of the social body as a whole.

Similarly, while participants' discussions of HPV biology linked to ideas of inherent machismo in Mexican male biology, couples' social responses to HPV positivity reflected the notion that good men could resist innate urges in order to perform companionate responsibility. Spouses in successful companionate relationships did deliberate social work, from research to emotional conversation, to frame HPV as just another health problem. Further, they used their explicit decision to see the virus in that light as a way to perform mutual support and emotional intimacy. Yet study participants in marriages that failed to meet current ideals of fidelity and intimacy saw the ideas about male biology featured in common explanatory models of HPV as reflective of husbands' problematic behavior. The virus seemed to them like a logical outcome of men's failure to live up to the new ideal of companionate responsibility. This was especially true as their understandings of viral risk being something that impervious men foisted onto vulnerable women mirrored the social risks of problematically "traditional" masculinity in which men's sexual behavior caused emotional harm to long-suffering wives. Failing to protect women against viral risk thus represented a larger failure to meet the long-standing cultural calls to advance the Mexican populace toward modernity through desirable gender and health behavior as discussed in chapter 1.

These widespread cultural assumptions about the linked biological and social natures of Mexican men were often implicit in participants' discussions of their explanatory models. The notion that "Mexicanness" innately predisposed men—figured as mestizos struggling with problematic masculinities inherited from both conquistador and Indigenous ancestry—to harm women lurked just under the surface of these discussions of viral biology. This assumption is what made participants' understandings of sex-specific HPV transmission and harm make sense. The importance of these ideas of innate but problematic gender roles became explicit when participants talked about the social consequences of HPV, which they related directly to ongoing social critiques of machismo in both their assessments of the meaning of positive diagnosis for their own marriages and their explicit discussions of masculinity analyzed in the next chapter.

FOUR

CULTIVATING COMPANIONATE FAMILIES

Ideals of Companionate Family

It is impossible to understand people's lives, marriages, and research experiences without also thinking about their experiences of reproduction and
how those also relate to changing ideals over time. Like being married, being
a parent has long been normative and seen as central to identity and social
belonging in Mexico (Ortiz-Ortega et al. 1998). In fact, people often value
reproduction even more highly than marriage. Having children can be a way
for people who have not followed other social norms to claim legitimacy and
respect. For instance, female sex workers might highlight their identities as
mothers to claim respectability, despite their stigmatized profession (Kelly
2008). People in Mexico have long experienced the family as the key social
unit, even amid changing economic and cultural contexts and a resulting
shift in emphasis from the extended to the nuclear family in urban, middle-
class mestizo life (Esteinou 2005).

Since the Mexican Revolution, people have been encouraged to act out contemporary ideals of modernity through their ways of parenting. Government education and health programs addressed women and men as mothers and fathers, tasking them with physically and morally cultivating ideal future citizens (Stern 1999). This has come to include consciously curating one's family size using birth control, which became a marker of idealized, modernizing mestizaje, in contrast to vilification of Indigenous people as uncontrolled reproducers holding the nation back (Soto Laveaga 2007). Historically, parental roles have been heavily gendered. Women have been seen fundamentally as mothers (Ávila González 2017), even when they act in public arenas such as the workforce (N. Sanders 2017). In turn, mothers have been understood as primary parents, echoing traditional divisions of gendered labor and the Catholic Church's veneration of self-sacrificing motherhood, while fathers were expected to further state goals of modernity within their families via provision and patriarchal leadership rather than care work (Joseph et al. 2001; Melhuus 1996). Elite and popular cultural portrayals of fathers, especially lower-class and Indigenous ones, have often framed them as doomed to failure at those goals due to the lack of will to overcome innate machismo, leaving women as the pillars of families (Bliss 1999).

Today, reproduction and parenting remain key sites for people to act in "modern" ways, which now reflect companionate ideals. Worldwide, "good" and "healthy" parenting have become ways to assert middle-class status and address broader social ills (Bertone 2017; Dermott 2012). In Mexico, collaborative work developing a small, well-tended family by using methods such as contraception and assisted reproductive technologies is a way to assert elite status, good citizenship, responsibility, anti-macho gender ideology, and idealized mestizaje (Braff 2013; Gutmann 2007; Singer 2017).

This ideology explicitly departs from "traditional" expectations that women should be maternal nurturers in emulation of the archetypal figure of the Virgin Mary and that men should demonstrate virility and masculinity by fathering children (Castro 2001; Melhuus 1996). Yet these new expectations have not fully displaced those prior ones. For example, assumptions that Mexican mothers are fundamentally responsible for domestic care and naturally self-sacrificing are built into current medical practices, from decision-making about organ donation to childhood obesity intervention (Crowley-Matoka 2016; Saldaña-Tejeda 2018b). However, emotionally engaged coparenting by mothers and fathers has also become a key feature of Mexican ideals of companionate marriage. This ideal links emphasis on child rearing as the heart of family life with calls for emotional intimacy and rejection of machismo as cornerstones of "modern" masculinity and family life.

For instance, spouses often extended their valorization of open communication, discussed in chapter 3 as a hallmark of companionate marriage, to their ideals of parenting. This was the case for the nurse Lola and taxicab driver Benjamín as they debated whether the human papillomavirus (HPV) harms men. After Benjamín noted, "If you want to stay married, don't stop talking," Lola explained that this approach extended throughout their family interactions: "We always talk, to develop a solution, even with the kids, about what we're doing. . . . We don't give the kids ultimatums. We just talk before giving them permission." For such participants in the Human Papillomavirus in Men (HIM) study and their partners, engaging in self-consciously open family communication was a marker of modern companionate marriage and parenting, which also served as a hallmark of higher class and educational status.

Of course, just as with spousal relationships, how people actually defined and practiced companionate parenting varied widely. Further, while engaged fathering increasingly has been seen as ideal and normative for several decades, that does not necessarily mean that couples who practice it espouse egalitarian gender roles (Gutmann 1996). Building on the discussion in chapter 3 of how couples incorporated the experience of HPV diagnosis into their performances of companionate marriage, this chapter moves up one level of scale to investigate how spouses sought to use men's HIM participation to enhance the health and well-being of their nuclear families.

Like the broader Mexican adult population, most HIM participants had children, and they frequently raised the topic of parenting in our interviews about their HIM experiences. Their narratives revealed the centrality of their identities as parents to their understandings of who they were as people and spouses, as well as to their daily-life decision making, including about men's medical research participation. They often described their children as the most important people in their lives and parenting as their most important duty. For instance, the Instituto Mexicano del Seguro Social (IMSS) physician Pablo (whose wife's ire at his failure to mention what he saw as insignificant test results was discussed in chapter 3) said that he and his wife's children "are the suns, and we're the planets that revolve around them."

Following participants' lead, here I analyze their HIM-related experiences as family events. I discuss how caring for and developing intimate relationships with children was a key life goal for the vast majority of HIM participants and their partners. Whether the HIM study was a major or a minor part of participants' lives, many saw participation as reflecting or enhancing their ability to be good parents. I first discuss participants' common understandings of their parenting goals in relationship to the HIM study. Then I expand on this discussion in case studies of parents discussing their interrelated HIM experiences and life and health goals for their families.

Just as spouses understood their own bodies to be interrelated within a joint couples biology, they similarly saw the family body as an interconnected unit in which one member's health directly influenced the physical and social well-being of other members. They understood the HIM study as furthering this goal in various ways, such as helping parents stay healthy to ensure that they could care for children, offering possible medical advances to children themselves, or serving as a source of sexual health care information that parents could share. Parents also saw these actions as ways to develop emotionally intimate and open relationships with children that extended the ethic of companionate communication from spousal to parental interaction. They drew on the HIM study as one of many life experiences through which they could teach and model this behavior. Thus, contrary to bioethical assumptions about medical research as an isolated event, many participants understood it—like any other life experience—as a potential resource for good parenting. In this way, participants' and their partners' views of what the HIM study offered reflected their understanding of biology as collective as they sought to "live for" others—in this case, their children—though varied daily-life pursuits, including HIM participation.

Incorporating HIM Experiences into Parenting

BEING HEALTHY FOR YOUR KIDS

Spouses often understood men's HIM participation to facilitate their material and social care for their children. For instance, they frequently described HPV testing as fulfilling what a salesman called a broader "obligation you have to be healthy for the kids." The IMSS warehouse worker Reynaldo, quoted in chapter 3 about learning how HPV can affect women, explained, "If I'm in good health, I know that in a given moment if there's any emergency, . . . I can take care of my people. If I'm well, as a consequence they'll be well. . . . They'll be calm." Alfonso, the construction worker (see chapter 2), similarly understood HIM participation as one of his and his wife's many health-maintenance practices. He explained that they engaged in self-care "for my daughters more than anything. . . . If I get sick, if something happens to me . . . , it will happen to them. I still haven't finished my, you could say, duty of raising them."

Such participants understood maintaining their health as a collective good with familial-level health and social consequences. They appreciated the testing offered by the HIM study because it helped them to fulfill their perceived moral duties as parents. This was the case for the driver Javier and homemaker Francisca, who saw both men and women as HPV carriers (chapter 3). While neither had HPV symptoms, both identified being healthy for their children as a main reason for HIM participation. Francisca explained, "If we're positive, we'll seek treatment, because I want to be healthy for my babies."

Being healthy for one's children was a virtue that some participants even sought to live out before conception. A publicist said about her husband's enrollment in the HIM study:

> I like that he's involved in this, because we're thinking about having a child. It's something that you need to plan. Of course, any woman at any time can have a kid, right? But I would like, or we would like, our baby to be planned and for us to be ready. And if we have something or he might have something, [participation in the study] provides the opportunity to know and take action about it, to avoid affecting our baby.

By contrasting their careful planning with imagined accidental pregnancies, she claimed a moral high ground, a modern parental outlook, and an implicitly higher class status by engaging in thorough preparation for parenting that included her spouse's participation in HPV research (see, e.g., Braff 2013; Singer 2017). Her comments reveal that participants and their partners saw their understandings of family members' well-being as physically and socially interconnected as a virtue in itself. By contrasting herself with others who do not consider how their own health can affect their children's bodies and life chances, she asserted that such a perspective was not universal but was held by those people with the mindset needed to have the best and most modern families.

HIM BENEFITING CHILDREN

In addition to enhancing children's well-being by helping to ensure the health of their caregivers, many participants expected their research participation to create medical advances that would directly improve their children's health. Although HIM was not a vaccine study, many participants discussed the development of new vaccines as a possible benefit to their children. For example, Javier said, "These little ones will benefit from those vaccines, and that's great." In an interaction that demonstrated his linked desires to support health advances and perform emotionally engaged fathering, he then turned to the toddler he had been bouncing on his lap and asked, "Right daughter? You like vaccines a lot?" as she cooed and reached toward him. Like HIM participants who brought spouses to their clinical appointments, parents who brought children to our interviews were both revealing their deeply intertwined daily life routines and biological fates and engaging in practices that created emotional closeness.

Participants also sought to model health-care use, and thus benefit their children's health by encouraging them to engage in preventative health care. For instance, Javier and Francisca treated their study visit as a family outing, bringing their young children to see their father engaged in health-related activity. He said that because his ex-wife had a uterine problem that she attributed to HPV, which she blamed him for transmitting, he had decided to join the study to try to ensure his and his present partner's health. Bringing their children made this aim a family affair, demonstrating how caring for one partners' health could be interpreted as care for the family unit in several ways, biologically and socially: by providing simultaneous opportunities for shared leisure, open communication, and learning about the value of health care. Participants not only saw spouses' and children's bodily fates as interlinked; they also understood their body practices to relate directly to the social practices such as intimate emotional sharing that they saw as hallmarks of the companionate family.

INCORPORATING HIM INFORMATION INTO SEXUAL EDUCATION

Parents often incorporated their HIM experiences into ongoing daily life efforts to teach children to care for their health, especially by providing sexual education, which they hoped children would use to avoid sexually transmitted infections (STIs) and unplanned pregnancy. Participants frequently framed the HIM study as a source of information that they could then pass on to their children. This was the case for the homemaker Guadalupe, quoted in chapter 3 about her belief that being a "carrier" was different from having HPV. Guadalupe was under medical surveillance after the discovery that she had HPV-related precancerous cervical lesions. She said that she hoped to join a proposed women's HPV study to gain knowledge that she could use to help her daughters avoid the disease. She believed that research participation would help her "to know about this topic because I don't know anything. I know that the little bit they've been telling me I can use to help my daughters. If they can avoid [HPV-related cancer], I want them to avoid it." Through such hopes, parents figured their own knowledge as directly protective for children's HPV risk. Information gleaned from the HIM study became a shared family resource rather than an individual attribute.

These efforts at sexual education fit into parents' ongoing attempts to mitigate a range of risks to their children's health, including the dangers posed by rising crime, through open communication explicitly framed as health education. Benjamín and Lola incorporated HIM-derived information and his modeling of self-care through study participation into a broader range of such educational efforts. For instance, they discussed seeking to protect their two daughters by teaching them how to be safe—for example, by avoiding drugged drinks. Benjamín said, "I always tell them, 'Look, daughter, if you go to a party or a dance, your soda, always take it with you or throw it away. . . . Don't let anyone bring you an open soda or an open beer, because there are many untrustworthy people."

They integrated such teachings into broader advice to perform what they saw as modern gender norms to cultivate well-being. They discussed the importance of teaching their daughters to take care of themselves—for example, by feeling empowered enough to refuse drinks from others. They linked this education to their emphasis on supporting their girls in achieving careers that would provide for them and obviate the need to rely on men. In our final interview, Lola voiced disgust with parents who say about their daughters, "It's OK if she doesn't want to study. To me, it's better that she marry." Finishing each other's sentences in a speech they appeared to have given many times before at home, the couple added that they tell their daughters that "the best inheritance we can give you" is encouraging you to focus on your studies and "see you working in a good position" to be economically self-reliant.

Despite their progressive politics, Lola and Benjamín gave advice that was tailored by gender in ways that reflected the cultural tropes of vulnerable women and dangerous men that were apparent in people's explanatory models of HPV. While their education of daughters emphasized protecting oneself from harm, Benjamín characterized his advice to his nephews in more active terms—for instance, exhorting them to "be prepared. There are rubbers everywhere. Buy some, because you can get a sickness. Get with it. Care for yourself enough. Don't take drugs because in the future, because with that vice . . . you can get killed."

Finally, by educating children about risks related to sex and violence, parents also performed the emotionally open and involved parenting that had become a local ideal and marker of modernity. Many used the practice to assert difference from their own, more traditional parents. For example, a business executive criticized her parents for never teaching her about sex and said that, in contrast, "I talk with [my kids] all the time . . . [even though] sometimes we start touching on things that embarrass me. . . . They're growing and developing, so they have more contact with sexual issues, drugs, the security problems in our country." Parents thus often incorporated HIM-derived information and experiences into broader daily-life efforts to model and transmit modern health and gender attitudes. They hoped those attitudes—together with their own efforts to stay healthy to care for their kids and to contribute to medical advances—would bolster their children's health and well-being.

Creating a Family Different from Unmodern Others

These efforts to care for children though education and parental provision contributed toward many couples' overall projects of creating self-consciously modern and companionate families. Their narratives regarding their cultivation of these types of family show that they understood themselves in part through a relationship of contrast to problematically unmodern others. By identifying themselves as different from families that reproduced sexist divisions of labor and machista ideologies, they sometimes implicitly and sometimes explicitly claimed higher educational, class, and racial status than those they ascribed to such others.

For example, Lola and Benjamín devoted much of our time together to discussing how they taught progressive gender norms through example, including by modeling equitable distribution of household duties. This included the examples presented earlier and inhered in the fundamental ways they structured their time and labor. Lola worked nights and Benjamín's schedule was flexible, so he took care of preparing their daughters for school, transporting them, and doing much of the housework. They contrasted their way of life with that of Lola's sister, who they thought was raising her son with macho attitudes.

They recounted that, while the sister and her family were visiting from Chicago, their eleven-year-old nephew ordered his sister around and told Lola, "In my house, I'm in charge." Benjamín said that he intervened in this sexism, telling his nephew, "Here you listen to my wife." The couple partially blamed the influence of his Guatemalan father for their nephew's attitude, saying that machismo was on its way out in Mexico but still thriving in Guatemala. The explicit intent of their critique was to demonstrate their difference from, and disapproval of, "traditional" gender roles. Yet their attribution of machismo to heritage from a country viewed as less developed and more Indigenous than Mexico also highlighted the racialized nature of such critiques. They implicitly contrasted an aspirational Mexican mestizaje, which entailed a behavioral and bodily whitening away from indigeneity, with the regressive gender practices from a country to the south framed as poorer and more backward.

Paty, the nurse, and Mario, the bartender, were also explicitly committed to living out progressive gender norms in their marriage and parenting. They, too, rhetorically grounded their efforts to raise teenage sons who would be "different" from other men in the family's difference from other groups whom they saw as insufficiently modern. This included the difference from other Mexican men that Mario discussed the desire to cultivate in chapter 2, and Paty's desire to be different from the women who enabled it. For instance, she noted that a man's equal participation in housework "depends on your partner, your wife has to let you help."

Mario and Paty reported transmitting these beliefs to their teenage sons by modeling equitable distributions of labor in the home. They explained that Paty did less domestic work because of her more rigorous employment schedule, while Mario transported the children to school and did the bulk of the daily housework. His transportation role became increasingly important over time: by our third interview, the couple felt that increasing violence made it unsafe for their sons to take public transit to school. Their sons also took on a share of household chores; by our second interview, the youngest had developed an interest in cooking and had taken over preparation of the family meal on Saturdays. The parents proudly discussed the influence that their sons' household participation had on their personalities and ideas about gender. Mario stated, "Now they know how to cook a little, sweep, mop, iron—that is, understanding that there are no machos in the house." Paty voiced their belief that this had shaped their sons' characters, adding, "And above all they've been inculcated with respect, equity, equality. That is, not yelling, not insulting, not using obscenities." They understood their modeling of egalitarian task sharing and respectful, intimate marriage as directly teaching their sons a progressive form of companionate responsibility.

They further saw these attitudes and practices as setting them apart as a modern, and thus implicitly mestizo rather than Indigenous, family. Mario noted, "Here in Mexico it isn't very common that the man does housework, prepares food, washes clothes. But little by little, we're getting rid of that taboo." Paty framed this change as a sign of progressiveness, adding, "Obviously, there are still marginalized towns where a six-year-old boy still acts like the boss of the house. . . . But at least here in Cuernavaca, I've seen a lot of change." The term "marginalized" is frequently used in press and government reports to reference groups and areas that suffer structural economic disadvantage, often conceptualized as Indigenous and rural despite the widespread poverty that also exists in urban centers (see, e.g., Fuentes 2013). Thus, Paty's comment positions her family at the front of the vanguard leading the mestizo population away from the problematically traditional ways associated with indigeneity and rurality, toward the future. In keeping with this vision of forward movement, Mario and Paty proudly located their own family histories on a progressive timeline away from the gender ideologies associated with rurality and indigeneity. They explained that they were proudly carrying on family traditions by raising their sons to think progressively about gender. Mario recalled the other residents of the small town where he grew up thinking it odd that the men of his family did "women's work" such as laundry, but that, as mentioned in chapter 2, his father had taught him to reject sexist divisions of labor. Paty added, similarly, "My parents were very dedicated to the idea that everyone had responsibilities in the house. . . . Even dad washed dishes, made the salsa. . . . We were raised like that, and obviously that's the same culture that we're leaving to our kids." For couples like them, raising companionate families reflected a proud commitment to social justice. Yet it was a commitment sometimes voiced and conceptualized in ways that reified the class and racial building blocks of Mexican inequality.

Diverse Family Experiences

ALMA AND JOSÉ: USING THE HIM STUDY
TO SUPPORT FAMILIAL WELL-BEING

Alma, a homemaker and seasonal day-care worker, and José, a worker at a wholesale company, incorporated information from the HIM study into their ongoing project of cultivating open communication with their children, which, they hoped, would enable them to avoid sexual and health risk. When we met, the spouses were both thirty-five years old and had a thirteen-year-old son and seven-year-old daughter. Unlike most HIM participants, they did not have IMSS health-care coverage, and finances were a constant difficulty for them. In fact, their economic situation deteriorated over time to the point that, by our final interview, they had moved in with Alma's mother in an attempt to pay off credit card debt. Yet they faced these problems with the explicit determination to stay "united" as a couple and family, seeing difficulties as "tests" that they could pass by remaining committed to their main value of open and communicative couplehood and parenting. They demonstrated this openness in our interviewes. Both were relaxed and talkative. José noted, "I could talk all day if you let me."

Over the course of these interviews the couple discussed the ways that they incorporated HIM experiences into their self-consciously companionate family life. They saw clear benefits for their children in José's HIM participation. Both expressed that they felt obligated to care for their own health to be there to support their kids. José said, "It's a responsibility—a huge responsibility—to have a family and children, so if they're offering the opportunity to live a better life and be healthier, that makes it much easier, right?" He characterized the HIM study as "an opportunity we could take to know what we had and combat it." This was part of "do[ing] what we can to give [our kids] a better life and to be with them" as long and healthily as possible. Alma agreed as she discussed her decision to join a planned but ultimately unrealized women's HPV study. She said, "I've always put my children first, and it's for them that I'll lose all day tomorrow here [doing intake for the planned women's study]. I come for them because they need us as parents, because we're the pillars of the family."

Alma and José were happy to take advantage of additional medical tests, such as bone density screening, which the HIM study sometimes offered as a courtesy to participants and their partners. They then incorporated the results into daily-life health behavior such as dietary change. For instance, Alma said, "[José] brought me the results from the study—for example, the ones about calcium. He said, 'You're low on calcium. We're going to, for example, drink less coffee. We're going to put more milk in. We're going to eat more cereal.' . . . The studies have helped us try to take care of ourselves a lot more." José saw this as an opportunity to redress some of the health problems he believed he had developed from his childhood, when he "had a less balanced diet because there weren't the economic resources." He said that he "used to ignore" the health issues he knew he should deal with because he lacked the resources to address them. However, his HIM test results and interaction with study staff had shown him that "there are lots of things that once you know about, you can do more [healthfully]." He framed this self-care primarily as a way to ensure that he could provide economically and emotionally for his family, but he also saw it as a broader social good. "It's a responsibility, as a human being, that I have to care for my health" to avoid unknowingly spreading disease, he said.

Since José and Alma did not have access to IMSS health care and had limited resources for private medical treatment, they also saw the HIM study testing as supporting their family by providing the couple with free health care that enabled them to focus their spending on their children. José explained that he would always choose feeding his children over paying for his own medical testing. But since his kids also needed healthy parents, he said, "When they gave me the opportunity to do these studies, I said perfect, great. I have to take advantage of this opportunity because sometimes I want to do [medical studies] but I don't have [the money], and in this case it won't cost me anything." José called the HIM study "a real support" because "if a test costs me a hundred pesos, and I have two children that I need to spend on so that they can eat, then in that aspect, now I'm thinking more of my kids than of myself, my state of health, although we know it's important. Would I first take care of myself and let my children go hungry?" So the free HPV and other testing HIM participation offered enabled him to maintain his own health without taking resources from his children.

The couple also saw self-care in general, and HIM participation specifically, as ways to model positive behavior for their kids. Alma noted that she had been "taught to teach by example." José added, "We have two children, who will also be parents some day or have partners, and we've thought a lot about that. If we don't give them a good example, I can't say anything to them about their behavior if mine is bad." Thus, José characterized participating in the study as "killing two birds with one stone: one is our health; the other is demonstrating how to live well." For them, living well entailed self-care, as well as open familial communication about a range of topics, including the health and life problems that could come from sexual activity. Alma lamented that "many families really lack communication," and José often discussed the importance of talking honestly about family issues to "live a happy life" together. Through such engagement they hoped to make their children feel "accompanied" rather than alone.

The HIM study enabled José to model sexual health care and to further open lines of communication with their children about sexual health. Alma's and José's parents had not discussed sexuality with them. In contrast, the couple deliberately used tactics such as discussion of HPV to relate differently to their own children. José said, "We don't want our kids to make mistakes because of lack of information." Alma added, "We try to be very open. We never want it to be like before. My parents never told me anything." Framing frank familial discussions of sexual health as a hallmark of modern, engaged, and responsible parenting, Alma discussed their efforts to "team up" with their children's teachers to provide sexual education. Her discussion of their efforts at sexual education also revealed it to be a forum for modeling progressive masculinity and parenthood. She said she told her son, "It's good that you go with your dad, that you and he discuss it like men and talk. Always remember that we've already been down this road. It's a well-traveled road that you're going down. We've gone down it. What you're living, we've lived."

The couple saw the HIM study as a resource for information they could share in these discussions. José explained that he valued information from trusted sources: "I'm a person who doesn't like to not know things or to come up with things on my own. I want to learn something concrete from people with experience, so I can be certain it's correct." They saw information from the study as highly trustworthy. Alma noted, "I've appreciated that the study has taught us how to defend ourselves and to defend our children against unwanted contagion." José similarly believed that the study "has helped us a lot, both as a couple and as parents," by providing sexual health information and increasing their comfort level with understanding and subsequently teaching it. After several years in the study, he said, "Now we don't feel shy about being able to express these things, to talk about them."

The spouses made direct use of HIM documents in these efforts. Unlike most participants, José even shared the medical reports he received from the HIM study with his son. "I have all my papers from this study, and I've shown them to my son," he said. "I say, 'You can catch this. [This is] how to avoid it.'" He planned to do the same with his daughter when she was a bit older. Both José and Alma reported sharing both personal and general information from the study widely. Alma explained,

> It isn't just our son [we share the information with]; it's also our daughter, our nephews, our whole family. . . . My son says, "Oh, mom, you already told me that. You're always telling me the same thing." But at least he has it engraved on his memory, that he always has responsibilities, and the consequences he can encounter if he does things he shouldn't do, without protection, without asking for information. Now he can't go in with his eyes closed.

In this way, the couple used HIM information as a resource to teach their children and others about how to prevent STIs and to help them grow into informed adults who would act in "responsible" ways.

For José this continued a lifelong habit of gathering and sharing authoritative knowledge about how to "live well." He had done military service at eighteen and enthusiastically discussed the adult education classes it offered, including instruction on "how to live married life . . . domestic violence, the topic of alcoholism, the topic of sexually transmitted diseases, [and] the theme of how you could have a good family." He recalled enjoying being given homework assignments about those topics from a workbook, which he felt enabled him to understand these important issues better. In fact, he had saved those educational materials, sharing them with Alma and then, later, with their fifteen-year-old son. José saw HIM study results as a similarly clear source of shareable information, noting that he liked receiving lab results because "it's something concrete."

In addition to modeling openness about topics such as sexuality for their children, Alma and José sought to cultivate and model a companionate romantic relationship. Despite the economic and time pressures they faced, they put deliberate effort into their love life. Alma explained, "We've had little time, with the kids, house, jobs—but a couple without intimacy isn't a couple. It's important for your well-being as a couple." José agreed, noting that partners who were unfulfilled might begin to look outside the marriage for satisfaction. To prevent this, he said, "We worry about the family, but also ourselves. We don't forget that. It's important for a lasting marriage." They saw their own happy romantic relationship as providing stability, comfort, and a path for their children to follow. Alma said,

> I think what's important is to raise our children well—so they understand how to have a good relationship, so they're not afraid to talk about things. As a kid, I knew my parents had lots of problems. I don't want my kids to have that. With my kids, if they want some cookies or candy, recently I have to say no, we can't afford that now. But they know that even without money, we're happy, living well. They know we won't separate. They have an image of us—not one that's perfect—but as their future, so that they can live a similar life.

So even when they faced an economic crisis so bad that Alma said it "made us feel sick in our souls," they consciously decided to face it collaboratively and, in José's words, "stay united." Alma recounted, "I told him, this is like a test for our marriage. If we get through this, it means we can get through anything worse. And we'll still be together, and, most important, together with our kids." She added, "We're the best models for our children. They see what we do and do the same." As a couple, Alma and José sought to use whatever resources they could—from medical tests to their own example of remaining connected despite adversity—to be engaged and supportive parents who instilled companionate and self-protective attitudes in their children.

MARTA AND ANTONIO: "MOTHER HEN"
PARENTS LIVING FOR THEIR FAMILY

Marta and Antonio were the participants who most explicitly voiced the concept of the family as a biosocial collective as they discussed their HIM study experiences. In our interviews, they talked constantly about their children and family life, presenting the ethic of living for one's family rather than for oneself as their explicit life philosophy. They had been married for twenty-five years, after meeting while they were both clerical workers in a Mexico City IMSS office. After Antonio transferred to a Cuernavaca clinic, Marta took an early exit package from the IMSS and, she said, "dedicated myself to the home." When we met, the forty-eight-year-old spouses had two sons, age twenty-one and fifteen, living at home.

In our first interview, the couple explained that all the decisions they made related to the need to care for their family. Antonio said, "I tell my wife that now I don't just think of myself, but in what I bring with me, which is her and my children." In fact, he described marriage as "unit[ing] our lives." Marta added, "My father had a saying he would tell us, that when one marries, your life no longer belongs to you. It belongs to your husband or your wife." She continued, "When you have children, then, again, your life isn't yours. It's your children's." She added that this interdependence "obligates you to think before exposing yourself to things. . . . I tell [my sons] always, always, always think about what we want for you. Think about how much we love you. . . . However difficult the situation, we're here for you." So the couple understood themselves not as individuals but as parts of an interconnected whole and sought to teach their sons to think similarly.

This understanding of decision making as reflecting one's moral obligation to live for one's family influenced Antonio's entry into the HIM study. The couple discussed the opportunity and saw it as a chance to get extra health surveillance while helping others. They framed the information he would get from the medical study, as well as the interviews for my project, as ways to perform the open communication that they valued. For instance, after our first interview Marta thanked me for giving them the opportunity to know themselves better by talking together about their experiences.

They also discussed Antonio's medical research participation as an action that set him apart as a man who lived up to ideals of responsibility, marital intimacy, and progressive masculinity. He recounted, "I signed up, and then they asked me to invite friends at my office." However, he said, "They didn't want to do it"—perhaps because they hoped to conceal their "sex lives and activities" from their wives. Contrasting himself with his colleagues, he said, "But I, with my wife—thank God we have that communication between the two of us. Since we met, we've been, apart from just being husband and wife . . . , we've been a stable partnership." Antonio's HIM participation thus became an arena for performing, and modeling, the interdependent relationships that they believed set them and their marriage apart.

They were also proud that their marriage emphasized companionate interaction among all family members. Marta explained, "Our goal as parents is for the family to be united," so they prioritized communication, openness, and shared recreation as a family unit rather than as a couple or individuals. When I first asked her to describe their marriage, Marta answered by focusing on the family as a whole. She said, "Our family situation is really family-oriented. It's most about spending time with the boys. We have two sons. Now they're big—one is twenty-one, and the other is fifteen—and we try to guide them. We're *papas gallinas* ('mother hen' parents), really closely engaged. I don't like them to go out in the street much. I prefer that they be in the house."

While this focus on spending time together inside the domestic space reflected fears of violence and negative outside influences on their sons, it also highlighted the parents' desire to live as a unified group. For instance, they saw the parental bed as a site for emotional engagement as a family rather than sex or respite. When their younger son became fearful about the growing violence, they responded by encouraging him to sleep together with them. Marta said happily, "We were like the three little pigs! . . . He slept in between us, even though he's much taller than us!" The couple also saw this closeness as setting them apart as good parents. Antonio contrasted their actions with those of the parents of the pregnant teenagers Antonio encountered in his IMSS clerical work, who, he believed, had a low "cultural level." Marta added that this lack of culture affected "the level of care that parents give." The couples' deep engagement with their sons was thus also a way to claim educated, middle-class status.

Antonio and Marta did not find their son's presence in their bed disruptive because it meshed with their focus on emotional exchange rather than sexuality. Both spouses defined ideal marital intimacy in terms of companionship, not carnality. When Antonio discussed their relationship, he emphasized that they had begun as friends and preserved their ability to talk through any issue. Marta described their sex life as "very healthy" precisely because it came second to companionship. She described it as "maybe not so frequent. We're based in, our marriage is based in spending time together, which is even more intimate. . . . We have other ties than carnal ones, more emotional, more as being together as humans. I married a great friend . . . and that's served us well." This included backgrounding sex in favor of foregrounding care for children. As an example of their commitment to health and family, Marta proudly noted that after she became pregnant, they did not have sex until their babies were more than seven months old. They saw directing their energy and care to family rather than couples' needs or individual desires as the right way to live.

They sought to model this lifestyle for their sons. Marta explained that they always thought through their actions—including their spousal interactions—in terms of what their children would learn from them. She said, "We try not to argue in front of them. We try to be good models for them. Examples teach better than anything else." After the couple went jointly to several of Antonio's HIM appointments, they decided that it was also a good opportunity to model self-care and openness. They brought their younger son to our final interview so he could participate and experience communicating about medical and life experiences. Marta said, "There's no other recipe for success than communication." This sharing about the HPV study experience fit into their broader project of educating their sons about sexual risk and protecting them from harm.

They proudly discussed teaching their sons responsibility through caring surveillance. For instance, Marta recounted,

> I use washing their backpacks as a pretext, and I take everything out in order to see what they have inside. . . . Fortunately, I've never found more than wrappers of candies and sweets they weren't supposed to eat. But for example, once I found a condom in one of their bags, the eldest's. . . . He said, "Mom, they gave a talk [in school] and handed them out." And I said, "You know, they'll spoil if you leave them in your bag." I explained not to carry them in the bag, or pocket, or wallet; that you have to treat condoms specially.

Antonio also visually inspected his sons' genital hygiene when they became teenagers to ensure that they were caring for themselves properly. These actions intentionally broke barriers of privacy and individuality to teach about sexual health in a way that supported Marta and Antonio's philosophy of living for others. She described deliberately teaching her sons the family philosophy of interdependence, saying that she had told her older son, "OK, you're going to go away to university . . . , but remember that your life isn't just yours. It's mine, and you have to care for it as if it were mine. And that makes him think a bit before exposing himself [to risks]."

While Marta and Antonio's emphasis on emotionally open family interaction reflected their wholehearted embrace of the self-consciously modern ideal of companionate marriage, it did not reflect explicitly progressive gender roles. Marta discussed "inculcat[ing] my sons with a lot of respect, for women, and that they have to respect everyone," and Antonio often remarked how much he valued his wife's advice and wisdom. With Antonio working and Marta dedicating herself to the domestic sphere, their emphasis on respect linked "modern" ideas that all family members were emotionally equal with a "traditional" division of gendered labor. Further, they mixed expectations for their sons' gender performance that could be defined as traditional and modern. Marta policed her sons' gendered self-presentation, telling her eldest that "being modern doesn't mean getting a tattoo or a piercing. . . . If you pierce your ears, I'm putting a skirt on you." However, she and Antonio wholeheartedly embraced their younger son's academic focus on fashion design, giving feedback on his sketches and talking proudly about his participation in a bathing suit design contest. While they were unfazed by his interest in a pursuit that was not traditionally masculine, they expected both sons to conform to expectations of heterosexuality, marrying women and raising families. This expectation reflected powerful cultural expectations of the life course, as well as the couple's assumption that their sons would live for others, as they had been taught, replicating their family of origin and living well as an interrelated unit rather than as individuals.

ABEL AND BLANCA: BINDING TIES DESPITE BAD BEHAVIOR

Failures at building such cohesive relationships can also reveal people's beliefs about the nature of family interrelatedness. While the couples discussed previously sought to enact self-consciously companionate forms of family as a way to care for their collective biologies, Abel and Blanca's case shows how people might understand family bodies to be affected by problematically "traditional" gender performances and lapses of care. Their experience reveals how belief in the biosocial bonds among family members can serve to keep people related—in some ways, trapped—even as members of the family fail to uphold their social obligations. It also shows how such family members can use a shared belief in fundamental familial interconnectedness to make claims for emotional inclusion and belonging despite bad behavior.

Abel was a forty-four-year-old former taxicab driver who had been employed only intermittently since he injured his back in a car accident. He held court in our interviews, rapidly narrating his family's lives and difficulties, particularly his own failings and the need for his wife and three young adult sons to forgive them. He clearly valued the HIM study in part because of the attention it provided. My study further offered an audience with an attentive researcher, as well as his wife, Blanca, whom he alternately wooed, shamed, and apologized to as he narrated their experiences from his perspective. This use of our interviews highlights that they were a social forum in which participants created context-specific, and sometimes quite strategic, narratives that were revelatory of their interpersonal relationships. Pleading his case for a place in their family despite his infidelity and inability to provide support, Abel said that he had made Blanca and their children "suffer" greatly but was on a course of change.

The couple were as different in demeanor as they were in looks. Abel was whip thin, while Blanca had rounded cheeks and curly hair. A forty-year-old homemaker who had supported the family by selling catalog goods since her husband's injury, Blanca tended to sit quietly as Abel pontificated, modeling the forbearance promoted by her evangelical Christian faith. She rarely responded to questions, despite Abel's frequent exhortations for her to "speak up" and "talk openly" because sharing one's feelings was healing. Yet she was also not one to be bullied. When pushed to exasperation by what she considered lies, she concisely but vehemently disagreed.

Abel framed the story of their more-than-twenty-year relationship in terms of Blanca's suffering. He said that "it hadn't been easy for her" from the start. Laughing, he told me that he "stole" from her home in the State of Mexico. He convinced her to move to his home near Cuernavaca, where she got sick on the bus and was stung by a scorpion on her first day. Abel later added that he had fathered two children with another woman during their marriage, a fact that came to light when the woman sued him for support. They had also struggled economically, especially since his accident; they were one of the few couples in my study who did not have access to IMSS health care. Overall, Abel said, "My behavior hasn't been great. I cheated on her. I used to be a drunk. . . . I've done many atrocities to her, but she supports me a lot. She deserves a good life."

Abel cast his bad behavior in terms of both adherence to negative and divergence from positive masculine expectations. Blaming his infidelity on an inherent but problematic Mexican nature, he explained, "I'd been accustomed to women and drinking. Mexican men are macho, egocentric like that." However, he claimed to have matured out of such behavior after his accident. He continued, "I almost died. Now we have peace. I give the woman the place she deserves. I'm not a child anymore." Yet despite his claims to fidelity, which Blanca saw as outright lies, given continuing evidence in text messages from other women, Abel dramatically performed guilt for failing to live up to the provider role. For instance, he said, "I tell her, I'm bad because it's my obligation to provide for [*mantener*] the house. I say that if I can't bring in money, I won't even eat a tortilla." Blanca responded with exasperation that she never complained about his eating, suggesting she saw his hunger strikes as childish attention seeking. She also highlighted his lack of resilience, saying, "I don't doubt that the pain [from your injury] exists, but everyone has pain. You have to move forward. You can't live crying."

Such comments reflect how Abel's selective performance of emotional openness also contributed to his failure to achieve masculine ideals. He transgressed traditional masculine expectations of emotional closure by being dramatically vocal about his own suffering and feelings of guilt and shame. However, he also failed to engage in the emotional support and mutual sharing with family members that characterized the ideal husband and father in the modern companionate family. He recounted, "She says I'm like a candle in the street and darkness in the house. I do favors for anyone, and that bothers her. . . . She says I do everything for others; nothing for us." Abel saw his wife and sons as a cohesive unit that joined forces to shame and judge him. He complained that Blanca's critiques were echoed by their oldest son: "They always agree about everything. It's like she's Batman, and he's Robin. They say I should be home with the family."

Yet their criticism was not the same as exclusion. Abel characterized families as fundamentally interrelated entities in which members' actions determined others' experiences, characters, and fates. He related his immature behavior to his abusive upbringing, saying, "I had no childhood, only aggressions, humiliations. Now, I told my son this, now at forty-five all the stuff I kept in, I'm letting it out—all that I didn't get to do as a kid." Conversely, Abel cited refocusing on his relationships with his sons rather than his parents as something that enabled the behavioral change he claimed in our third interview. He said that thinking of his sons had enabled him to become more mature and thus avoid divorce. He explained, "I think of them before fighting, or before doing something dumb, and I stop."

Abel also discussed the ways that his and Blanca's relationships with their sons had fundamentally affected the children's characters. He praised his sons for developing emotional and physical health despite trying circumstances. He said proudly, "My sons don't look for fights. They don't drink or smoke. They're really healthy people." Demonstrating his belief in the enmeshment of the family unit, he saw this not simply as the result of his wife's competent mothering but also as a consequence of his sons' relationships with both parents, including his negative example. He explained, "I tell people that their rectitude comes from her. I tell them, take the good from me. If I come home drunk, learn not to drink. If I smoke, learn not to do that."

Considering this upbringing, Abel said, "The kids have always been very respectful. They've never failed me." He also stated that his other family members "have good values. I have no words to describe her and my sons. They've acted like a real family, and I'm paying for my errors." This payment came in the form of their clear dislike for him. Yet even as he failed to provide support and care, womanized, and threatened repeatedly to leave and sleep under a bridge or starve himself, he maintained the sense that he was a fundamental part of an interconnected family. While the members of the "real" family achieved positive emotional interactions of which he was not a part, he, even as a "bad" father and husband, remained inherently interrelated to and influencing of the others. Abel maintained that whatever happened, "We function. As a family, we function, with highs and lows."

Given his experience of interrelatedness, Abel was able to benefit emotionally from the successes of sons whom he also described as profoundly angry at him. For instance, he told me, "The oldest is twenty-two. He's a Jehovah's Witness. Everyone respects him, like his mother." Tearing up, he added, "I'm proud when people speak well of him. . . . The whole world admires him, respects him. It makes me swell with pride when people talk about him. It makes me feel—it elevates me . . . because my ego is fed when they talk to me about my son." Attributing his sons' goodness to both Blanca's positive example and his own negative example enabled Abel to experience his son as an extension of his own ego.

Like Marta and Antonio, Abel held the belief that family members should live for one another. While Marta and Antonio taught this perspective to their sons to encourage healthy and morally upright behavior, Abel also used it as a way to assert that he had a place in his family despite his bad behavior. Promoting the ethic of living for family, he recounted telling his sons, "Life hasn't been easy. I've tasked them with [caring for] their mother, because they have to look after their mother. Why? Because she's seen to you, cared for you, she's given you life, and if someone deserves respect, and if someone deserves that you care for them, it's your mother. Look after her. Dedicate yourselves to your studies; work up the energy to strive to be something in your lives so that someday you can pay her back."

In this comment, Abel articulated mutual care that promotes health and gives life as the biosocial interaction that constitutes a family. As he continued, he also inserted himself rhetorically into this web of mutual care and obligation. While he admitted to his failures as a father and husband and said that they justified his emotional exclusion from the family body, he also used such comments to claim belonging. He accomplished this by applying guilt to those that would marginalize an injured and flawed but well-meaning man. These comments further enabled him to perform belonging in the family by providing care—albeit via proxy—to others by directing his family members to care for one another. He continued, "I—it doesn't matter if I live or die—but yes, I want you to fight for her . . . because in reality she's the one who carries the household because I don't work. . . . Because of my health condition I'm very limited."

Abel also used HIM participation to make claims to both modernity and health behavior that provided care for the family biology, and thus to frame himself as deserving his place in a biosocial unit that he had previously affected only negatively. While enumerating his past failures, he made increasingly vehement claims over the course of our interviews to have changed his ways. He asserted, to Blanca's disbelief, that he had become faithful, variously due to his accident, his family obligations, and knowledge from the HIM study, which, he said, "opened my eyes. I saw that I wasn't living well, I could get AIDS, HPV, and I'd give them to her who is innocent." He used his negative HPV test results to assert moral goodness, saying, "Thanks to this program, I'm a clean person, with the security of knowing that I'm healthy." In these ways, he asserted that he had become a protector of their couple's biology, rather than someone who harmed the family biology by failing to provide material and emotional care.

He also made claims to morally upright modernity through participation in the HIM study, which he contrasted with assertions of Blanca's backwardness, to highlight his importance to their family and to shame her into staying. After discussing the benefits of medical research participation, Abel contrasted his views with those of Blanca, whom he said, "didn't want to come." He characterized Blanca as "the enemy of doctors" who never sought self-care; he, by contrast, described himself as a "messenger" for sexual health testing and decried the antimodern attitudes of people in rural towns such as theirs, where people "don't have education." In a dig at those such as Blanca who sought solace in religion, he said such people avoided testing in favor of the belief that "God will take care of me." Goaded out of her silence, Blanca retorted that government programs had given educational talks in their town, so now their neighbors were "not so ignorant." Voicing belief in couples biology, she also explained that she did not need to be tested for HPV: "If he's clean, I am."

For Abel, claiming modern health behavior and familial care through HIM participation was one variation on a broader rhetorical strategy he used to justify his place in the family. He alternated between praising Blanca's long-suffering persistence in their marriage and blaming her backwardness for their problems. For instance, when I asked Blanca, "Why did you stay with him?" she replied, "Honestly, I don't know." Abel took back the conversation, saying, "You know what I think, doctor? She's with me because she had an old-school upbringing [in which] divorce is a sin. Her mother died; her father is old. So she can't move back home and has nowhere to go." She protested angrily, "I have places I could go." He interrupted, "Rural education [to] respect your husband." He continued with a shift to praise, saying, "She's a very noble woman. I have to wash my mouth out to speak of her. If there were a word higher than 'saint,' she would be it."

Abel's discussions of family cohesiveness and interrelatedness despite his masculine failings, and his calls for emotional inclusion by family members he had wronged, reflect his and Blanca's shared understanding of even unhappy families as biosocial units. For Abel, a family ideally included emotional acceptance of and support for one another, on top of their inescapable interrelatedness. He noted that his wife and sons had "acted like a real family, despite the grave way I failed them." He also said that, by failing to meet his obligations, "I haven't acted like a real father or a real husband." This, he said, meant that it would be the legitimate "consequence of my actions . . . if tomorrow my wife or sons run me out of the house or hurt me, because they're right. I failed them." Of course, he said this in a tone suggesting that only a bad family member would actually take those technically appropriate actions.

While Abel thought a "real" or ideal father and husband would care for his family, he nevertheless asserted the belief that he, Blanca, and their sons were inevitably biologically and socially interconnected. This was demonstrated by his account of his children adopting healthy behaviors by learning not to copy his bad ones, as well as by his ability to feed his own ego with praise received by his sons. He told me, "I feel proud because I know that [my sons] don't have vices. They're not people I have to worry about. I know that if I go to work, they'll be watching out for their mother and their grandfather. So in that sense I'm grateful to God and to this life for the family that in reality I have." Ultimately, he painted a picture of family members ideally living for and accepting one another but fated to fundamentally influence one another no matter how badly they behaved. Participation in the HIM study and our interviews enabled Abel to make a rhetorical appeal for emotional inclusion, based on assertions of modernity and behavioral change, in a biosocial unit to which he would belong even if he "ran away to starve."

The Family Body

In this chapter, I have discussed the main ways that participants and their partners incorporated HIM experiences into broader life projects of developing companionate families. Just as spouses often interacted about study events in ways deliberately intended to demonstrate open, intimate communication in their marriages, they also incorporated HIM participation into ongoing efforts to develop similarly companionate relationships with their children. Participants and their partners sought to create self-consciously modern forms of family in which parents cared deliberately for a manageably sized family unit by meeting family members' physical and emotional needs. In parenting this way, spouses also acted out norms of middle-class mestizo respectability and followed long-standing calls in popular culture to advance the nation through such comportment. For HIM participants and their partners, caring for children in the modern ways associated with those class and ethnic statuses meant not only providing material necessities, but also providing psychological support for children's growth into modern, responsible adults. Parents understood a key part of this support to be education, ranging from instruction about how to be safe and healthy to modeling happy marriage, open communication, and self-care. The HIM study became one of many resources on which parents drew to realize this ongoing life project.

While such companionate family relationships have become ideal in many world regions, in the Cuernavacan context they reflected culturally specific ideas about the nature of relationships among family members. Just as HIM couples understood their biologies to be fundamentally interrelated, they believed that both their bodily states and their parental actions directly influenced their children's health and well-being in the physical as well as emotional realms. Parents understood men's participation in research to support the entire family's health in a variety of ways. They believed that HIM checkups would help to ensure that parents were able to care physically for children; used HIM participation as a way to model health-care participation and open communication that could help children to deal with physical and psychological problems; incorporated information they learned in the HIM study into sexual education; and hoped that HIM-related medical advances might protect their children from HPV-related harm. These views were exemplified by Alma and José's commitment to using medical research as a way to support their own health and education so they could allocate health-care resources and health-enhancing knowledge to their children. These understandings represent context-specific takes on emerging strategies parents worldwide use to provide care in precarious times shaped by new biological harms and opportunities, from cord blood banking to modeling resilience in the face of environmental danger (cf. Cho 2020; Santoro and Romero-Bachiller 2017).

The majority of research participants who had children talked frequently about them in our interviews as they answered questions about their marriages, lives, and HIM study experiences. This reflected the importance of children to people's lives in general, and the local cultural emphasis on being as parent as a crucial aspect of being a full person. It also demonstrated the ways that family interactions in daily life provide constant opportunities to put broader ethical projects into practice (cf. Kremer-Sadlik 2019). Beyond representing locally specific takes on these widespread experiences of parenting, the presence of children in parents' discussions of men's medical research experiences reflected their fundamental view of families as collective biosocial entities. Many shared the ethic, so clearly articulated by Marta and Antonio, of "living for one another" rather than living for oneself. This philosophy overlaid a specific understanding of biology: that family members' bodily health fundamentally influenced not just the emotional or life experiences, but also the physical well-being, of other family members.

I argue that these perspectives reflected family-level application of the cultural understanding of the Mexican national body discussed in chapter 1: the idea that the health and well-being of the physically and socially interrelated mestizo populace could be advanced through individual practices of modernity. People's incorporation of HIM experiences, which focused clinically only on men's bodies, into varied aspects of family life demonstrates their broader understanding of families as collective biologies in ways shaped by this national ethos. From that perspective, people's efforts to be good and modern parents through HIM participation and other activities were simultaneously practices of social and health care for the family unit. The next chapter focuses on how people extended such efforts to the Mexican populace as a whole.

FIVE

CREATING A "CULTURE OF PREVENTION"

Self-Care as Civic Engagement

Participants in the Human Papillomavirus in Men (HIM) study often saw themselves as uniquely positioned to advance the Mexican national body through their individual health behavior. While everyone in the study felt economically precarious, given the recent financial and instability crises and long local history of inequality, many participants were relatively privileged. Since the HIM study recruited largely at the Instituto Mexicano del Seguro Social (IMSS) and a few major local companies, participants were often highly educated and held stable professional jobs. Others who lacked these advantages were drawn to the study by an interest in health care or a search for creative ways to support their families. Thus, the HIM participants and their partners were an aspirational group who understood themselves in contrast to both an imagined backward and indigenized poor and a corrupt and irresponsible elite. Participants often saw themselves as the vanguard who could lead a society composed of these groups forward.

They thought of themselves as educated and modern enough to model ideal health and gender behavior for others, but poor enough to be untouched by the corruption they thought plagued rich politicians and oligarchs. Those who worked in state health care and education especially saw themselves as tasked with what they explicitly called "changing the culture" away from both ignorance and corruption. Later I discuss the common cultural and historical threads on which HIM participants drew in their reasons for the relatively uncommon decision to participate in sexual health research as a way to live ethically.

Their belief that they could effect change through medical research engagement drew implicitly on a long history of public health calls for people to rise in racial and class status by engaging in self-consciously modern health behavior. As discussed in chapter 1, postrevolutionary public health campaigns have tasked a Mexican populace framed as mestizo with nudging their families and the nation forward by modeling modern hygiene and comportment (see, e.g., Bliss 1999; Joseph et al. 2001; Stern 1999). Given this history, it is common today among implicitly mestizo-identified state health workers—such as those represented in the HIM population—to see their role as educating patients they see as backward or overly Indigenous about modern health practice and self-presentation (Smith-Oka 2012). This same population continues to see their own health behaviors as representing and advancing social progress (Braff 2013).

They are thus engaged in locally specific, racialized versions of the identity projects through which middle-class people worldwide seek to maintain status and affluence, despite increasing economic instability and unreliable or dwindling state care for citizens. Social scientists have identified two main trends influencing middle-class behavior. One is the adoption of individualistic, entrepreneurial attitudes as a way to seek wealth and demonstrate modernity amid increasing privatization and decreasing state provision of resources (Cahn 2008; Freeman 2014). The other is understanding themselves as representing universal or ideal social values to support the existing systems of power that have privileged the middle class, even as those systems falter (Sumich 2016).

The HIM participants and their partners incorporate both trends into their behavior in a unique way inflected by the cultural trope of a biologically and socially interrelated Mexican populace that should be aided by the Mexican state but is not identical to it. By engaging in medical research, HIM participants supported the postrevolutionary state's constitutional goals of care and advancement for the populace by promoting modern health and gender behavior, even as the government itself faltered amid insecurity and corruption. Many also did so by serving as proud and faithful workers in state health and educational institutions, even as they critiqued government corruption and inefficiency. In a context where the "slippery" state unreliably lives up to its promises of provision (Crowley-Matoka 2016), they also entrepreneurially used medical research participation to secure high-quality health care. They saw their own enhanced health as directly benefiting others in the social bodies to which they belonged, from their families to the Mexican populace.

The ideology of collective biology specific to such ideas about Mexican-ness contributed to participants' context-specific take on the middle-class responses to precarity emerging globally. In worldwide contexts, from diseases to disasters, promoting prevention through personal risk management has become a strategy for shifting the expectation of care from the state to the individual. A version of this neoliberal ideology is sometimes promoted by Mexican elites. For instance, the anthropologist Susan Schneider found that state health officials in Morelos used critiques of poor patients' "culture of ignorance" to blame them for their own ill health and to justify the creeping but controversial privatization of aspects of the health system by promoting an ethic of individual over collective responsibility (Schneider 2010). Yet in contrast to those health officials—as well as to middle-class contexts worldwide, where people understand individualism as the path to modernity and upward mobility—HIM participants hoped that their own personal pursuit of health care could start a positive ripple effect for the broader Mexican populace.

Middle-class HIM participants, too, used the language of culture change, often saying that they hoped to model a "culture of prevention" to counteract the "culture of ignorance" that led many Mexicans to avoid health care. However, I argue that their calls for cultural changes in health behavior took on a collective rather than individualistic meaning because they understood themselves to be biologically and socially interlinked with others in the Mexican social body. Rather than espousing individualism or justifying privatization, HIM participants incorporated their own preventative practices, in which they included medical research participation, into explicit efforts to enhance collective well-being. They reported hopes of inspiring modern health behavior in more "ignorant" members of the social body while enhancing population health by caring for themselves to better care for others. They thus saw individual health behavior as affecting not only themselves, but also the collective biologies to which they belonged. Further, these actions justified demands that the government live up to its promise of care by supporting a project they saw as state-sponsored science.

The metaphors that participants used demonstrated their views of themselves as the parts of a broader whole that would be influenced by their own preventative activities. This was put poetically by the IMSS physician Pablo, who described his children as the sun around which he and his wife orbited (see chapter 3). He also discussed himself as part of a mathematical aggregate when talking about his hopes that his HIM participation would help others. He said, "Someone has to be a positive statistic ... if we want good results" that can help future generations. Similarly, Javier, the driver, said that HIM participation was a way of "contributing" to society and described himself as one "little grain of sand" that could create change together with many other people behaving well in the metaphorical beach of society.

Further, participants saw themselves as those parts of the societal whole best positioned to advance others. They often described themselves and their family members as *sano* (healthy) and *limpio* (clean) in terms of their behavior and attitudes, as well as their physical bodies. For instance, participants called everything from fidelity to noncoercive marital sex "clean" behavior, which they listed as a cause of physical health, including human papillomavirus (HPV) negativity. Parents also called dutiful children whom they believed avoided drugs, crime and sexual exploration "clean," as when Marta and Antonio, the "mother hen" parents" in chapter 3, bragged that their sons were "good, clean and honest." People also discussed their pride in modeling "healthy" marriage for their children and others. Their view of individual health and cleanliness as contributing to the aggregate character of the social body reflects long-standing discourses of individuals as representatives of a biocultural Mexican whole hoped to homogenize toward progress in part through the performance of progressive hygienic behavior.

The HIM participants and their partners thus used medical research participation as a distinctly middle-class, mestizo Mexican form of "biological citizenship." This is Adriana Petryna's (2003) term for people's use of emerging identities based on membership in biological categories to claim rights from their government and assuage unmet needs. Engaging in medical research became a way for people associated with the HIM study to assert modernity and biological and behavioral "health" and "cleanliness" that they believed positioned them to advance their society, despite crisis and state fragility. Being a HIM participant involved obtaining and promoting state health care. So participants implicitly justified their critiques of the "slippery" state, and their calls for enhanced state provision, by showing themselves to be good citizens who illustrated the need for modern services by making use of them. Their hope that these individual actions would have consequences on the level of collective, as well as their own individual, biologies was a hallmark of this version of biological citizenship.

Participants saw themselves as citizens of two entities: the Mexican state and a Mexican social body interlinked by race and culture. Although those entities were separate, their fates were intertwined as the state influenced the social body by providing or failing to provide care. This situation reflects the complex realities of citizenship in precarious contexts worldwide. While officially framed as a binary status that someone either has or does not have, citizenship in practice is a spectrum on which people can access varying degrees of rights based on their social status and self-presentation (Petryna and Follis 2015). In keeping with this complexity, HIM participants and their partners used medical research participation as a practice of citizenship in both of these arenas. They sought to advance the mestizo social body from within by modeling modernity. By using state offerings to accomplish this, they called on the state to live up to its promises of support for that body.

In this chapter I discuss how participants and their partners framed HIM involvement as one of many daily life activities through which they performed and modeled self-consciously modern gender and health behavior in the hope of promoting population advancement, as well as critiquing the governmental failings that they feared would thwart it. I argue that people drew implicitly on cultural narratives of individuals as parts of a national biosocial whole to engage in a particular form of biological citizenship, where they sought to aid the Mexican populace directly through their own behavior as members of a middle-class vanguard, drawing, but not depending, on state aid in these efforts.

I begin by discussing how people used participation in the HIM study as a way to modernize Mexico by both "supporting science" and deliberately attempting to promote a "culture of prevention" over one of "ignorance." I then expand my analytic lens to other daily-life arenas, contextualizing people's HIM activities in the wider range of work and political and social activities through which they attempted to promote modernity in the social body while coping with state failings. I deepen this analysis in an extended case study of retirees from the state health system, who actively sought to do this in arenas that ranged from medical research participation to dance competition. By identifying the relationships among participants' hopes for medical research and their other daily-life forms of civic participation, I show how middle-class people drew on understandings of a mestizo collective biology to enhance population health through their own actions while calling on the Mexican government for aid rather than promoting an ethic of individualism. Thus, while they focused on individual health behavior in ways that, on the surface, looked similar to the "everyone for themselves" ethic of neoliberalism, HIM participants hoped that their acts of individual risk reduction would aid collective biologies.

Supporting Science

Study participants hoped that their support of science would help future generations in several ways. They expected that the research findings they helped to produce would yield new treatments from which their children's generation would benefit. They also hoped that supporting the local practice of science would help to create a modernity-oriented society that valued and promoted scientific inquiry and medical care for its people. Finally, they sought to promote these values by modeling pursuit of community welfare. This was the case for Javier, who discussed his expectation that daughter and other children would "benefit" from medical advances generated by the HIM study (see chapter 3). Javier also used his participation to model modern self-care by bringing his family to appointments. He opined, "The study has been good in general terms. Sometimes it is a bit of effort to come from [his nearby town], but as they say, we do this not for an individual benefit but for a general one. To help many, right?" From this perspective, HIM participation was an act that was worth personal inconvenience because it would enhance the health of the populace.

The taxicab driver Pedro felt similarly. He said he joined the study to "support science" and "help future generations," in keeping with his desire to advance both himself and his society. He contextualized his interest in medical research in his more general ethos of aid, saying, "I look for a way to help" in every aspect of his life. This included in the home, where he sought to share housework in a performance of modern masculinity: "I look for ways to help: wash dishes, sweep." Pedro cast himself as the starting point of broader change, saying that, for a healthy society, "You have to start with yourself, at home, eating healthy, exercising, going to the doctor." He took on this attitude when he enrolled in "self-help" classes during his military service. Pedro described with real pleasure how he had enjoyed doing the homework that guided him through reflection on how to be a good parent and spouse, how to be financially responsible, and how to care for one's health. He then described sharing this education with his wife, Carmen, a beautician. She said that Pedro's enthusiasm for personal development spread to her and sparked her own interest in medical research participation and preventative health care. They both articulated hopes that their new attitudes would spread to their children and beyond, making future generations healthier and happier.

Participants sought out diverse ways to support science and medicine to aid the social body. A few people became self-appointed spokesmen for the HIM study. The IMSS warehouse worker Reynaldo proudly wore a HIM polo shirt and said he told his colleagues, "It would be good for you to show up and see if you could be part of this project." Others extended the desire to use their own body to help others beyond the HIM study—for example, by donating blood. This was the case for the lab technician Jaime, who said, "If I can help—for example, if I can donate blood to the Red Cross if they need it—that's no skin off my nose. If I can help, well, good; and because of that, I've taken notice that many people suffer from ignorance and from fear and from shame." For him, such practices helped others not just medically, but also by providing a model for self-care, educated social engagement, and proper moral conduct.

Others emphasized the need to support scientific infrastructure both to help modernize Mexico and to provide care for their compatriots. Pablo raised and critiqued the idea that Mexicans were "Third Worlders," using vaccination programs and his research participation as a counterexample. He characterized himself as a "guinea pig" helping "to create a better quality of life for the coming generations." His wife supported this perspective, noting that research participation was a societal need. "Someone has to give their time," she said. Pablo concluded that his actions enabled them to "hope that for [future generations] there will be fewer problems with aggressive sicknesses such as the human papillomavirus." Through their support of government health programs, they both hoped to support the provision of care to others and made claims on the government to provide such care to disassociate their country from the "Third World."

Paty and Mario, whose efforts to model egalitarian gender roles are discussed in chapter 3, also saw local medical research as a key marker of modernity that enhanced government health-care provision. Paty said that, as a nurse, she knew about the local health research scene and found much of it lacking. "Many research projects that they do here are practically refried versions of what already exists elsewhere," she explained. In contrast, she saw the HIM study as cutting edge, both scientifically and because it broadened the scope of sexual health research to men in a way that supported progressive masculinities. The couple expressed gratitude that the HIM study had made men's HPV testing available locally and that it emphasized disease prevention—an attitude they found lacking in society broadly and IMSS offerings specifically.

Mario said that part of his motivation to join the study was to be in the vanguard of men getting tested. "That's also why I entered the project on HPV in men," he explained. "They told me that someone had to be the one to start it." Paty had also planned to participate in a study of male HIM participants' female partners. The couple saw that study's cancellation due to lack of funding as evidence of Mexico's failure to modernize. Mario related the cancellation to corruption, saying, "It's a shame, it's really a shame for our Mexico, that, on the one hand, there isn't money to do really important programs, and on the other, a week ago they found that a former governor's house—or, rather, his secretary's—cost almost one hundred million pesos." Paty then linked that misappropriation of resources to Mexico's lack of progress in relationship to other nations:

> If our government continues with this mentality, the country will never be equal to the United States, like Canada, like some European countries. Look, Japan, that's so tiny. My God—it's doubling, tripling us in education. Talk about people who strive, people who want to get ahead.... You just have to see how Hiroshima looked after the nuclear bomb compared with Mexico. Years after, they've had so much change after that destruction, and Mexico keeps staying the same, destroyed.

By participating in research, Paty and Mario sought to support government programs that would aid the nation's development.

Similarly, María, a school administrator, framed research participation as a way to improve societal-level health and model modernity. When discussing her role as an educator regarding students' health, she said, "I think that the culture of prevention has to change in Mexico." She added that she had tried to inculcate this attitude, as well as help students to obtain preventative care, by inviting her student body to enroll in a national vaccine study following a local outbreak of dengue fever. These participants saw supporting disease-prevention research as a way to align themselves with positive national priorities, despite antimodern corruption and even lackluster science. Overall, people often saw medical research participation as directly benefiting future generations' health while supporting a cultural shift toward modernity and calls for government investment in science.

Changing the Culture

Reflecting their visions of themselves as part of a broader Mexican whole, people often cast changing their own behavior as an initial step toward modernizing the society at large. For instance, just as some men saw periodic HPV testing as an aid for staying faithful (as discussed in chapter 2), others believed HIM participation helped them engage in the modern health behavior they saw as valuable but not necessarily part of their enculturation. Reynaldo, the warehouse worker, noted, "One here [in Mexico] doesn't take care of oneself; one doesn't go to get checkups." However, he added, being in the HIM study "obligated me to be here [in the clinic], present, involving me in this role [of self-care] practically by force." He said that this inducement to get regular health care had also led him to get regular checkups for hypertension, which he had long known was necessary but was unwilling to do before becoming accustomed to regular medical contact.

People often framed their own personal development as having a ripple effect throughout their families and Mexican society. Since they saw themselves as parts of a larger biosocial whole, they believed that advancing themselves could positively influence the others with whom they were interrelated. This was exemplified by Vero and Alberto, whose efforts to modernize their marriage are discussed in chapter 2. Vero was active in a women's personal development group. Through readings, discussions, and group events, the group "teach[es] us to value ourselves as women, and . . . also teach[es] us how to act with the kids, the husband, the family." She felt that her self-esteem had been improved by learning that, "first, I have to value myself and love myself, in order to be able to give that love to those around me." Vero framed the group's emphasis on personal growth not as an individualistic self-improvement project, but as a way to positively affect those around her by improving her performance of ideally modern mothering and marriage. Vero and Alberto also engaged in several "self-help" activities for couples, which they saw as not only improving their own relationship but creating a ripple effect of positive change through their extended family. Both thought that Alberto's shift toward a progressive form of masculinity within their relationship had served as a model for his relatives. Vero noted that one of Alberto's "machista" brothers has separated from his wife. "They had all these problems in their dysfunctional marriage," she said, "and, well, he noticed you as an example. He told you, right? That he would like to live as [Alberto] did . . . a model to follow."

The HIM participants and their partners often explicitly hoped that by modeling modernity in such ways, they could turn the tide against a "culture of ignorance" that they believed was prevalent and that they thought had directly negative consequences for Mexican collective biology. Many participants decried the "ignorance" that they believed led their compatriots to avoid sexual health care and stigmatize those who engaged in it. This was echoed by the IMSS warehouse worker Jorge, who said that he enrolled in the HIM study after seeing the negative consequences, including divorce, that befell two of his male friends who contracted genital warts caused by HPV. Jorge was divorced and saw getting his sexual health checked out as a way to make himself a desirable partner in a hoped-for future relationship. Based on this logic, he took one recently divorced friend to the HIM study with him. However, he said, despite the havoc that inattention to his sexual health had wreaked in his friend's romantic life, the man dropped out after just two visits. "Ignorance is a cancer that has no cure," Jorge said, framing his friend as suffering from a willful *dejadez* (lack of self-care) that could extend out to harm others. In contrast, his own HIM participation served as a marker of the progressive masculinity he believed would make him a good partner.

Men like Jorge saw their HIM participation as evidence of their achievement of modern manhood, which they believed they could help spread in their society. For instance, Mario described such behavior as the way to "start a snowball effect." Research participants and their partners imagined this snowball growing to incorporate themselves, their families, and the Mexican population, fomenting behavior with positive health and social consequences that might counteract the harms of problematically traditional "ignorance."

This included the hurt caused to some by their "ignorant" relatives and friends. Ginebra, the homemaker who discussed her unexpected anger toward her HPV-positive husband in chapter 2, recounted a painful experience: she had told her cousin about her HPV positivity, seeking both solace and to spread the word that people should get tested. However, her relatives responded with by stigmatizing her: "I have relatives who knew what I had, that I had papilloma, and they didn't want me to use their bathroom because their daughters would catch it. It was so weird for me. I seriously wasn't allowed to enter their bathroom. I hadn't yet entered this program, but that attitude bothered me a lot, because it was discrimination." Ginebra said that researching HPV on the internet and learning through the HIM program "cheered [her] up" by giving her proper information. By seeking to educate her relatives about the true nature and transmission routes of HPV, she sought to feel less like a pariah and more like a member of the vanguard promoting modern health and gender attitudes over ignorance. She said that she hoped that "being participants in the study can advance education," turning others toward this modern orientation.

PROMOTING A CULTURE OF PREVENTION

As suggested by the language of combating ignorance, participants often discussed how they hoped their actions would shift "the culture" forward. People's understanding of Mexican "culture" as shared by a group also united by mestizo biology underlay their hopes that changing culture could directly enhance population health. They often explicitly discussed their desire to create a "culture of prevention" that would promote modern health and gender behavior—demonstrated by things such as men getting checkups— and thus also concretely improve the health of the Mexican social body. For instance, Leo, the IMSS clerical worker, said that the HIM study "is good because we [in Mexico] don't really have the culture of prevention." Beyond its impact on his sexual practice, he noted, participation in the study "was really good because, well, the appointments obligated me to go. They would tell me it was time, and I would go. . . . You never do that."

María, the school administrator, similarly said, "I think that the culture of prevention has to change in Mexico. Everyone has to get checkups every six months. General tests, to detect whatever problem. Then we can spend less on health, if everyone does those preventative tests—especially the kids, who are sometimes very vulnerable." She believed that such self-care would aid the broader society by freeing up economic resources, as well as improve the health of vulnerable groups. Her support of and engagement with her husband's HIM participation was one of many ways that she framed care on the individual or couple level as a way to enhance societal health. She noted, "I take good care of myself because if I'm healthy when people need someone to donate blood, I'm always able to participate. So one has to feel good, to be well. You have to take care of yourself to be able to do what is needed." Echoing the statements of parents caring for children through HIM participation, she saw her own engagement in prevention as benefiting a broader collective biology both directly, through blood donation, and indirectly, by serving as a model for how to live more healthily. For such participants, HIM participation facilitated the performance, maintenance, and social transmission of cultural attributes they viewed as healthy for the population. They hoped to foment a "culture of prevention" that would emphasize risk awareness and self-care as collective care, in contrast to what they viewed as a problematic local tradition of ignoring health problems until they became acute.

As these examples suggest, HIM participation was only one of the many daily-life arenas in which people sought to model and promote the culture of prevention. They often did this through other forms of routine health care. For example, a utility company retiree hoped that he could "serve as an example for the people around us, because they observe us also." He offered the example of his adherence to frequent checkups for a kidney problem. He said his friends' and relatives' mental health was improved by the removal of the stressor of worrying about him. He further hoped that his self-care would encourage them to get health-promoting checkups of their own.

While many participants kept their HIM experience fairly confidential, a few discussed it widely, serving as self-styled health messengers. This was the case for Abel, who used being a HIM study "messenger" to claim modernity and the moral high ground—despite his infidelity and unemployment (see chapter 4)—in part by contrasting himself with backward others who did not seek sexual health testing. Abel said,

> [Talking about sexual health] isn't difficult, including the experience I've had with human papilloma and everything they've taught me here. I dare to talk to people. That's what you have to do—dare to communicate to them. . . . So in one sense I'm a messenger. I try to help people learn that they have to be careful with these diseases, from human papilloma to AIDS. . . . So I talk to the people who are my neighbors, who work with me, or who I always hang out with about that topic.

For such participants, modeling or educating others regarding the benefits of self-care was a way to support national health and modernization through individual research participation.

MODELING MODERNITY AT WORK

The HIM participants and their partners also often saw the workplace as an arena for combating a culture of ignorance. This was especially common for state workers, who sought to promote cultural advancement not only by providing health care and education, but also by modeling modernity in the workplace in ways such as supporting meritocracy in place of advancement through corruption. In this way, they sought to directly shore up government services through their promotion of cultural change. For example, Paty said her work as a nurse helped her to do the modeling and education that everyone should be doing. "I think, practically speaking, we all need to do health promotion," she said, "because health education isn't just the job of a promoter or a nurse or a doctor. It's everyone's job." She also made explicit the class element inherent in such beliefs: "I've noticed that people's economic level, if it's medium [or] low in general, they don't want to get [vaccines], and those at the high level in general come and seek them." She compared that with low-income people's unwillingness to take advantage of free food supplements for their children and desire instead to "continue [eating] their Cheetos." Such comments framed HIM participants and their spouses as ethical actors and worthy models who could lead less-educated or -modern community members into a cultural shift that would benefit their health and the physical and social well-being of Mexican society.

Importantly, Paty hoped this cultural advancement would enhance, rather than supplant, government care for Mexican citizens. She critiqued her colleagues for often doing the minimum in their state jobs. She said her own striving to make a difference in patients' lives had caused conflict with those problematic coworkers. "Last year, when I was in another unit," she explained, "my coworkers [sarcastically] nicknamed me 'Saint Patricia' because I helped people a lot, even if I didn't have to." Despite this conflict with her work colleagues, Paty was proud of her commitment to going above and beyond in her work, calling herself "one of those people who really suits up for the game [*pongo la camiseta*]." She saw her nursing work as a site for modeling modernity for patients and colleagues to support the government system that, in turn, supported people's use of preventative care.

Workers in private industry also used their jobs to support collective well-being. Mario, Paty's husband, expressed similar feelings about his work as a bartender. While tending bar might, on the surface, be seen as the opposite of promoting self-care, Mario saw it as a professional job in which he sought to advance through training and proper state licensure. He took pride in modeling hard work and efficiency. He also left a well-paid position because he believed the management was engaged in criminal activity. Thus, while people's efforts to model modernity often focused on children or the domestic sphere, as discussed in chapter 3, participants including but not limited to state health professionals also identified paid employment as an arena for modeling a self-consciously modern work ethic and rejection of corruption and self-interest.

Beyond promoting modernity in their families and at work, HIM participants engaged in civic and political efforts to change the culture in ways that would promote what they saw as healthy lifestyles and forms of governance. Participants sometimes characterized the context of government corruption and increasing violence as a "sick" state of affairs that harmed everyone. This was true for the researcher Roberto and the school administrator Griselda (see chapter 3). Both worked in state institutions that they believed helped people. Yet they saw the government as a whole as corrupt and harmful. For instance, in our interview in 2011, they discussed their fear that fraud would change the results of the 2012 presidential election, as they (along with many others) believed had occurred in the defeat of the leftist candidate in the previous election. They planned not only to vote, but also to be involved in citizens' groups "watching the polling places . . . to ensure that there isn't fraud." They feared that their candidate would be sidelined by corrupt political actors, since "he is concerned with the well-being of the society, not personal interests," as Griselda put it. Like many other participants, they blamed corrupt politicians for the mounting insecurity crisis. Roberto said that the "narco-politicians" in power "watch each other's backs. It's a mafia. It's the worst era in the history of Mexico."

Griselda and Roberto linked this situation to gender and economic inequality on the local level, saying that Cuernavaca was emptying out as people fled crime and hardship. Griselda said, "We can't trust the police. . . . They're very corrupt and linked to the narcos. They're violent, they're ignorant, they're wild. In [the nearby town of] Jiutepec, we heard about two policemen who raped two lesbians, to 'make them women.' They're homophobic. It's a really sick thing. What we're living through is really sick." This metaphor of sickness reflected literal connections that participants often drew between national problems and the ability of health interventions to model a progressive way out of them—both for people in general and for agents of the government specifically.

While Roberto and Griselda focused on the state's inability to maintain transparency and safety and to support progressive ideals regarding gender and sexuality, others associated widespread insecurity with failures to protect children from harm. Rafael, the dental technician, expressed such ideas. He critiqued the government for poorly regulating tobacco sales to minors, framing this as a gateway to narcoviolence:

There's a lot of narcotrafficking, lots of drugs in the streets. . . . More young people are addicted every day. Today, with cigarettes, there were reports that kids between nine and eleven are beginning to smoke, and the society, the government isn't putting a stop to that. They keep permitting the sale of cigarettes to minors, even though it's prohibited. . . . Soon [the kids] won't want a cigarette. . . . Soon they'll go for other drugs.

Participants often saw HIM and their other civic practices as ways to combat this state of affairs. They sought to heal the literal and metaphorical "sickness" of the social body of which they formed a part, despite the government's failure to do so. For instance, after a series of comments that involved modeling responsibility through risk management—discussing liking to get medical tests to stay on top of his health and the warnings he gave his children about how to avoid violence—Reynaldo began to critique the government. Making explicit the relationship between these practices of care and the state's failure to protect citizens, he said, "We have to take care of ourselves. Here in Mexico, the authorities don't."

In addition to research participation, many participants were involved in other activities through which they self-consciously lived and modeled what they viewed as modern health and gender practices. As discussed in chapter 4, participants most commonly framed parenting as a key site for this cultural transmission. Some were involved in educational reform or engaged in heated critique of the educational system. Rafael critiqued the system as being "in favor of transnational businesses" such as Wal-Mart rather than serving the nation. He attributed rising violence partly to the fact that, given this misguided focus, "The authorities who oversee education at the national level are really wrong. They got rid of the books about civility, about civics, about etiquette." These statements directly followed his critique of young boys being inculcated with machismo, linking increasing gendered violence to national systems he believed served foreign rather than local interests.

Mario and Paty voiced another critique, characterizing national-level bureaucracies, including education, as "mired in vice" and indicting Mexican teachers as lazy and self-centered. They believed that teachers' strikes had worsened their children's education. "Yes, it's good to protest, but for the good of the country," Paty noted. "You need to know the difference." By supporting mandatory testing for teachers, Mario said, "We as a family are trying to [create] change, and we hope that more families will continue to unite in this." In these efforts they called for teachers to mirror their own efforts at aiding the social body: modeling modern Mexicanness and behavior as state workers, for the good of the social body and in the hopes of raising the quality of the "slippery" state institutions that served it. The HIM study was thus one of multiple life arenas in which people such as Paty and Mario hoped their actions would help others while inspiring a shift toward modernity in both the social and state bodies of which they were citizens.

Ricardo and Itzel: Modeling Prevention and Civic Participation

Ricardo and Itzel were a couple in their mid-sixties who had both retired from government health jobs. They exemplified the common aims of benefiting from and shoring up state infrastructures of care while modeling extragovernmental civic engagement to advance the Mexican social body, despite government unreliability. They were chatty and outgoing in the HIM study and beyond. At a restaurant where they took me to feed me "Mexican delicacies," they knew the servers by name and asked after their relatives and health. Both were slim and dressed formally in slacks, with stylish blouses for her and polo shirts, often topped with a HIM study baseball cap, for him. This dignified daily dress contrasted with the revealing sequined costumes that they wore in the photographs they showed me of their hobby as senior citizen dance champions. These varied forms of attire together reflected their personalities, which combined fun-loving civic engagement with a view of themselves as educated, forward-looking, and responsible for leading others toward similar behavior, despite mounting insecurity.

COMPANIONACY AND MODERNITY IN THEIR FAMILY

Ricardo and Itzel, who had been married thirty-eight years when we met, had been early adopters of companionate marriage. Itzel recounted that she had never planned to marry. She was an only child, used to independence. She had seen school friends marry and be unhappy. So instead of marriage she sought independence and self-determination in a nursing career. She and Ricardo met when he taught her statistics class. He "worked to convince her" that marriage to him would not compromise her goals, she said, and reflected that he had also benefited from her modeling of how to be an educated and modern person throughout their marriage.

They had two children: a boy and girl now in their early thirties who lived in other Mexican cities, were single, and had professional careers. The couple expressed pride that their children diverged from the local norm of living with or near one's parents into adulthood. They had encouraged their children to focus on work and wait to marry and said proudly that both, in Itzel's words, "seem to have less desire to marry with every passing year." They described emotional closeness with their children that did not depend on proximity, and Itzel spoke with horror about how people their age became shut-in babysitters for grandchildren rather than getting to enjoy hobbies. However, they cast these somewhat atypical attitudes as a modern version of Mexicanness rather than a break from their community. For instance, Ricardo recounted a Belgian friend of his remarking that she had not seen her mother for eight years. "I see my mother every eight days," he said. "That's one of the Latino customs. . . . It would kill me not to see my mother for eight years." He added, "The Anglo-Saxons have a different culture, but here we're very tightly knit." Thus, while their lives differed from the local norm, Ricardo and Itzel saw themselves as an ideally modern version of an innate Mexican disposition to closeness.

LEARNING AND PROMOTING PREVENTION

Along with respecting Itzel's emphasis on individuality within familial closeness, Ricardo said he had actively adopted the orientation to self-care with which she had been raised. In her middle-class family, Itzel recounted, "From a little girl, I had that education, and that's why I studied nursing. I think that if one has education, more education, well, you try to take care of yourself, because unfortunately, ignorance makes one neglect oneself." Ricardo had been born into poverty and said that he "didn't have that education as a kid." Instead, he credited his wife and colleagues in the Secretariat of Health, where he had worked as an accountant, for teaching him to "pay attention to the importance of self-care."

In our second interview, Ricardo discussed lingering pain from childhood injuries that his family had lacked the resources to treat. He contrasted his adult self with that upbringing, saying that he now actively sought care for these problems, because "we have the culture of health." Itzel added, "Of prevention." Ricardo explained,

> I worked in the Secretariat of Health, and there I realized the importance of self-care. My wife also induced me to try to care for myself, get checked out, and that's also why I've assumed this attitude. I didn't have that education as a kid. They raised me like the animals. . . . My economic situation was very humble, and they treated me with home remedies. But now that I'm older, I try to attend to the things that can help me have a good quality of life.

For Ricardo and Itzel, engaging in preventative care was both a wise activity and a marker of class status. It meant that one was thinking about the future, of both oneself and the broader social body, in a way they associated with modernity and responsibility. Ricardo said that his work made him "conscious, to have the culture of health in mind; it's better to prevent than to cure." For instance, he had quit smoking after his boss showed him a set of diseased lungs to scare him out of the habit. They saw preventative health care as a sign that one was educated and disposed to care for oneself in a way that would offer a high-quality life.

They also saw this promise of quality as extending beyond their own bodies. Ricardo viewed his HIM participation as a direct outgrowth of his adoption of a middle-class culture of prevention that could aid others who had not yet been convinced of the need for self-care. Like other participants, he cast himself as a part of a broader societal whole that could be aided by his enrollment in medical research. He called himself a both a willing "guinea pig" and source of "raw material" for research that could help other Mexicans. He and Itzel sought to participate in health research whenever they could. Ricardo said that at each checkup, "I ask if there's any research program that I can join."

This habit reflected both his understanding of himself as part of a broader Mexican social body and his desire to be different from its norm. For instance, discussing his hopes for a long life with Itzel, Ricardo noted that the average Mexican male life expectancy was seventy-three. "It worries me that the life expectancy of the man is less than the woman's, on average," he said, "but I want to break the record." Moving immediately from his individual to the social body, he concluded, "We men need to be careful of our health." The spouses thus saw the HIM study and similar activities as enabling them to monitor Ricardo's health while promoting the "culture of prevention" and the companionately responsible form of masculinity that they had championed as state workers. Ricardo summed this attitude up by saying, "I'm a person who likes to participate in programs that benefit health—individual or collective."

Beyond helping to generate scientific advances, they saw the HIM study as a way to improve the Mexican social body's health by spurring cultural change in people's attitudes toward health care and the problematically traditional gender ideologies that turned men away from it. He said that HIM enrollment was a "marvelous" opportunity to get checkups "that not many people take advantage of"—"because of ignorance," Itzel said, concluding his sentence. Both saw men specifically as being "more resistant" to seeking treatment and engaging in prevention. He said that discussions with their friends had revealed that men often "prefer not to know" what is wrong. Itzel added that that attitude was silly because they just get sicker but "could have prevented the disease." The couple saw their role as educated people as spreading their culture of prevention. They did this by modeling preventative care and research participation for others. For instance, Ricardo often wore his HIM study baseball cap. He saw it as affirmation that he had achieved status as a "loyal" and "interested" patron of health research, telling me often that he had been given the cap "for being a faithful client." Itzel also extended the work she had done as an IMSS nurse by continuing to do health education. She said that she frequently told others about their checkups and research participation, saying, "This is all beneficial for you—it would be stupid not to participate."

EXEMPLIFYING "THIRD-AGE" ENGAGEMENT

Ricardo and Itzel were particularly conscious of the need to maintain their health as they aged, self-identifying as "senior citizens" who could both enhance their retired life with efforts to stay healthy and model this for other seniors who, they thought, let themselves go in older age. They implicitly linked these efforts to the modern orientations to marriage, health, and civic engagement that they valued. For example, given both their happy marriage and ability to retire after well-paid professional careers, Ricardo said, their main goal now was to really enjoy "the years that are left of our lives" together.

They believed this required active engagement in their community, intellectually and physically. They read several newspapers online every day, seeking to stay informed of the news and educated about current events. They also sought out announcements for free local events and attended all they could, from movie screenings to environmental rallies. They also made extensive use of the retirement benefit of excursions and activities for pensioners from federal employment, going on vacations and attending lectures especially for "third age" (later life) retirees. "We're not those people who retire and sit around," Itzel said, with Ricardo finishing the sentence: "watching television, no." Beyond participating in such events, they incorporated small acts of civic participation into their daily lives. For example, Itzel made a habit of bagging the trash her neighbors left in piles before the street dogs could get into it and spread it around. Ricardo joked that Itzel hoped such displays of cleanliness would shame the neighbors into change.

In such ways, they lived what they saw as a modern and active older age while promoting their values to those around them.

The couple's involvement in competitive dance epitomized these goals. They had "caught the dance bug" several years before we met and participated in *danzón*, a Cuban musical style with a formal partner dance that had long been popular in Mexico, especially among seniors. They initially became interested in dance as a form of exercise that could help Ricardo's hypertension, but they also quickly came to see the intimacy and cooperation it required as a boon for their relationship. Ricardo called it "emotional therapy" and said that it that "helped him to get along with and better understand my wife." Itzel added that they had seen people their age divorce after a whole life together, because they had grown apart, and they sought to avoid that fate through shared activity. Ricardo continued: "When you have defects of intolerance, we need to try to forgive each other, to overcome that for a happier life, a healthier life." He said that dance forced them to do that: "If I'm mad, I have to calm down, because we have a date to dance together. She has to dance with me. We need each other."

Itzel and Ricardo had become deeply immersed in the world of danzón, traveling around Mexico and even to Cuba to participate in workshops and compete in the third-age category of dance competitions. In addition to aiding their intimacy and cardiovascular health, they said, danzón enabled them to tap into both the global present and the unique history and essence of la raza cósmica. According to Ricardo, danzón is "an amalgam of music from Africa, Europe, Latin America" that includes dances that run deep in the Mexican past, like those "our ancestors before the conquest . . . to music for the moon, the sun . . . , as well as erotic dances [that] scandalized Spanish royalty." The first things the couple showed me when I visited their home were their dance trophies and photographs from their dance-related travels. For them, the hobby connected all the attributes that they saw as important for their identities: cosmopolitanism rooted in a shared Mexicanness, community engagement as active seniors, preventative health activity, and family intimacy.

MODELING MODERNITY AMID INSECURITY

While Ricardo and Itzel emphasized the need to modernize their shared Mexican culture to secure well-being and prosperity, they also believed structural political and economic changes were needed to enable this shift. For instance, they saw their own relative economic security as the fruit of both their personal circumspection and government support. They both received federal pensions and expressed concern that they would be cut by a faltering government. However, Itzel noted, "Fortunately, we have the culture of saving, so we have a reserve in case something happens." She explained that she had been trained to save money by a father who "taught me to administer myself well." They expressed sadness that this habit was unusual, seeing an inability to save money as a fundamentally Mexican trait. Ricardo explained that not saving "is a debility that we Mexicans have." Itzel added, "Yes, especially the women. We like this; we like that. When there's a kid, we want everything for them. Thank God, I've never had that situation of not having enough to eat the next day." With these comments they located themselves as the modernizing edge of a Mexican populace that needs to grow out of innate profligacy, including that induced by regressive forms of gender and family.

However, while the couple believed that Mexicans as a whole needed to start "taking care of themselves" and "saving money," they also criticized the Mexican government and oligarchy for creating a structural context that made this almost impossible. Amid the increasing insecurity at the time of our second interview, Ricardo voiced disgust at an interview he had read with "Carlos Slim, the richest man in the world" and the highest-profile member of Mexico's power elite. According to Ricardo, Slim saw retirees as a "social burden" and "declared that it would be convenient if people retired after seventy because the population has a longer life expectancy." This flew in the face of his and Itzel's life course of acting out ideal citizenship through an active, state-subsidized retirement following dutiful careers in the federal health system. Insulted at being considered a drain on the country's economy, they shifted into a discussion of how government failures to address the rising violence had curtailed their earning potential. After their retirement, Itzel said, "For a long time, we worked. We were merchants, but we stopped doing that precisely because of the insecurity, because we would have to take our goods around, delivering them, and now that scares us." They saw government provision of security and care as a necessary condition for cultural adoption of prevention, which included entrepreneurialism.

Itzel continued by explaining how the violence had constrained their activities. She said, "Now we also don't go out to social activities at night, or we make plans but stay briefly then come back quickly because now after ten o'clock we're scared." They discussed trying to reconcile their desire to be actively engaged seniors with the mounting threats. While "older adult groups usually meet earlier," she said, "with the insecurity, well, we meet *way* earlier!" She laughed and continued, "Even yesterday we went to an event. It was from two to six in the afternoon, so it was still light out and, well, we try to take care of ourselves a bit more but still enjoy our dancing."

While they tried to remain optimistic, Ricardo and Itzel said that they found the insecurity draining. This was especially true after their daughter was mugged. While she waited for an early morning bus to work, men cut her purse strap to steal it and gashed her hand in the process. She was so frightened that Itzel went to stay with her until she healed, both physically and emotionally. The couple's son was a casualty of the crisis in another way: he lost his job as an architect in Los Cabos because North American investment in the area had dried up. Itzel concluded, "All the insecurity that we've been having, I feel that it causes exhaustion." Ricardo added, "This insecurity really has us upset emotionally, not just for our daughter, but for the situation this has our whole country in." Itzel explained, "Now, one can't live with tranquility," and Ricardo continued, "It affects your health." He said that he felt less able to deal with other stressors, such as the impending death of his own mother, because he was constantly upset by the rising crime. "It's a really bad problem for the whole population," they said, voicing their belief that the violence crisis was directly harming the social body's mental and physical health.

While they often called for Mexicans to overcome innate dispositions to avoid preventative healthcare and financial planning, they blamed the government for the current state of affairs. For instance, Ricardo quoted Andrés Manuel López Obrador—then the leftist presidential candidate and now Mexico's president—saying that the sum that would have bought fifty kilos of tortillas in 1997 would only buy five kilos today. Ricardo said that "basic needs" had gotten "more expensive, in a brutal way." By our third interview, he had developed a full critique of the government's failure to provide jobs and care for citizens as the main cause of violence. "How many people are unemployed? How many young people?" he said. "It's a Petri dish that the bad guys take advantage of. . . . [There's] a whole group of youths that are a lost demographic; most [are] not educated and don't have the opportunity to work. That leads them to focus on illicit activities." The couple also sharply criticized the government for its complicity in rising crime. "The government minimizes or hides the reality," Ricardo said, "to the point where now one doesn't trust the authorities." Itzel added, "Tremendous delinquency has infiltrated everywhere. You don't even know with the police. It's better not to tell them anything."

They continued to model a culture of prevention for others, engaging in what they saw as modern and desirable civic participation even as the world seemed to crumble around them. Ricardo said, "We try to meet bad times with a brave face"—for instance, by taking advantage of, and thus demonstrating the need for the government to offer, events for third-age federal retirees. "We still try to spice up our lives, looking for healthy diversions at prudent times of day," he said. Itzel added, "It's a really difficult situation. But we try to take care of ourselves and maintain ourselves with healthy distractions." Yet they also believed that meaningful change in the behavior of the Mexican social body was impossible without change in the government's ability to provide security. Itzel said that, while they still supported medical research, "We don't see these [health] projects really advancing until the government puts an end to this tremendous delinquency that has infiltrated everywhere." Their efforts to lead others in the mestizo social body toward a "healthy" life, despite the lack of a culture of prevention, were thus hamstrung by the government's and elites' failure to provide the security and economic opportunity that were a necessary condition for such change.

Promoting Health and Desired Selfhood—Individual and Collective

By combating government "sickness," "delinquency," and cultural "ignorance" through civic participation in and beyond health research, participants consolidated their own positions as respectably middle-class citizens while seeking to redress the problems plaguing their society. They crafted locally specific versions of the identity projects through which middle-class people worldwide seek to maintain status despite increasing economic instability and unreliable or dwindling state care for citizens: individual risk management and support for the ideologies and systems that had privileged them, despite their precarity. Participants in the HIM study and their partners combined these responses in ways that reflected their visions of themselves as members of a collective Mexican biology. They entrepreneurially sought out arenas, in the HIM study and daily life, where they could enhance their own well-being in ways also intended to promote collective health. They also carried on a long local history of governmental efforts to encourage gender and health behavior that would modernize and aid the populace, even as the state itself faltered. The hopes of participants such as Ricardo to simultaneously benefit both "individual" and "collective" health reified cultural notions of the nature of the Mexican social body and enabled them to assert privileged positions as its moral leaders.

Their adherence to the tropes of modernity that the state had long promoted also enabled Itzel and Ricardo to critique the government for failing to provide adequate care and security. States have often promised services to citizens in exchange for modern behavior, including adherence to idealized tropes of race and gender, then failed to provide resources, such as access to health care, that people need to live out these ideals (Charles 2013). In such contexts, people might self-consciously perform modern behavior in efforts to hold up their end of biopolitical bargains and thus encourage the state to do the same (see, e.g., Obrist 2004; Street 2012). They, individually or as part of groups, can also partner with faltering state institutions to meet shared goals while propping those institutions up (Gerrets 2015). As good citizens promoting a "culture of prevention," HIM participants felt justified in calling on the state to hold up its end of the deal. Those who worked for state institutions also sought to create change in their workplaces from within, modeling professional and anticorrupt provision of care.

Participation in the HIM study was thus an act of citizenship. Through it, people asserted themselves as a vanguard with the education and resources to identify and promote modern behavior, and without the "ignorance" they attributed to the poor or the corruption they believed compromised the Mexican elite and weakened state institutions. Further, participants and their partners used medical research to perform biological citizenship in two related but distinct entities. They sought to advance the mestizo collective biology that served as the metaphorical beach holding their individual "grain[s] of sand," which they could advance from within by being "positive statistic[s]." They also hoped to counter and critique the corruption of the Mexican state, which they saw as failing to live up to its implicit bargain to provide care for those who engaged in the national modernization project of mestizaje promoted since the Mexican Revolution.

Overall, medical research participation became one of many practices of civic engagement through which people asserted citizenship in this social body. They sought to advance it through their own actions as especially forward-thinking parts of that whole and attempted to lay claim to rights, such as health care, that the Mexican state unreliably supplied. Analyzing couples' participation in the HIM study alongside their practices of citizenship outside the clinic, from election monitoring to dance competition, shows how they were able to view the ostensibly individual experience of genital testing as a forum for fomenting broader societal change. Seeing themselves as citizens of both a "slippery" state and a racial group in need of modernization, they used medical research participation as one of many civic efforts to "improve the culture" amid the insecurity that threatened middle-class gains.

SIX

EVANGELICALS PARTICIPATING AS PIETY

Evangelical Christianities in Mexico and the HIM Study

Religion is an important part of people's everyday lives in Mexico. The population is overwhelmingly Catholic, and Catholic symbols are visible everywhere, from roadside shrines to decals of the Virgin de Guadalupe on buses. Though officially secular, public medical care in Mexico is similarly infused with Catholic ideology, as when the Virgin Mary's maternal suffering provides a model for how mothers should act when children require donor kidneys (Crowley-Matoka 2016). Catholicism is so taken for granted that, after a long conversation about how I was a Quaker-educated, atheist secular Jew with a Unitarian partner, a participant in a prior study concluded, "But you're Catholic, right?" However, many Catholics experience religion as a cultural and general ethical commitment without conforming to strict doctrine or attending regular services. When making life choices, including those related to gender, sexuality, and health, Mexican Catholics tend to interpret religious doctrine flexibly to support behavior they deem desirable based on secular discourses of modernity, including public health messaging (Amuchástegui Herrera 1998; Hirsch 2008). The majority of Catholic participants in my study discussed religion more as a social context than a spiritual endeavor. They mentioned marking religious holidays and life events with church attendance and took Catholic theology for granted, but they rarely discussed religion as a direct motivator for action in daily life.

In contrast, the small but vocal group of evangelical Christian participants in my study described all their activities and experiences, including medical research, as venues for living out their faith. They announced their religion almost instantly upon meeting, seeing their study participation, like all other life events, as a God-given opportunity to live piously and proselytize. They reflect a broader trend—in Latin America and worldwide—of people converting to evangelical forms of Protestantism in significant numbers. Protestant sects have grown steadily in Mexico since the 1970s (Dow 2005), and the 2010 census found that almost 13 percent of the Morelos State population identify as non–Catholic Christians (INEGI 2011). Locally called *Cristianismo*, evangelical forms of Christianity are increasingly visible in Cuernavaca, from the growing frequency with which the taxicab drivers I chatted with began to proselytize to the construction of the city's first American-style megachurch.

In this chapter I focus on the experiences of the four couples and three female partners of HIM participants who participated in my anthropological study and self-identified as Cristianos. They were demographically diverse, ranging in age from twenty-five to sixty, and worked in blue- and white-collar jobs both within and outside the formal economy. All were married, and all but the youngest couple had children. Cristianos were the participants most likely to ask me to participate in daily life activities with them, inviting me to attend church worship and related social gatherings. So in this chapter I contextualize my analysis of interview data with information from participant observation in those settings.

Focusing on Cristiano participants' experiences enables me to further the book's analysis in two ways. One goal of this chapter is to show how people incorporated the Human Papillomavirus Infection in Men (HIM) study into specifically evangelical versions of the kinds of efforts to live out gender and health ideals commonly discussed by study participants of all faiths. They include the idealization of companionate marriage structured through benevolent, non-macho patriarchy and familial closeness achieved through pious interaction, which I discuss in detail in the next section. This chapter investigates how participants lived out religiously inspired goals at the various levels of scale discussed in prior chapters, as well as at the additional levels of the church family or congregation, and their embodiment of spiritual relationships with God. The HIM study offered one of many daily life arenas for living piously by caring for one's God-given body, maintaining health by monitoring the wages of previous sexual sin, and supporting the companionate (if fundamentally patriarchal) marriage and masculinities that their churches promoted. I argue that participants' relationships to the HIM study were influenced not only by their spiritual goals, but also by their churches' emphasis on piety as embodied practice. So I discuss how they incorporated medical research experiences into ongoing efforts to perform *testimonio*—to live out the traits they also praised through prayer and evangelism—through pious health and gender behavior in daily life. Thus, mundane life arenas including medical research participation became sites for the embodiment of participants' spiritual goals.

Focusing on Cristiano participants' experiences also enables me to pursue a second goal in this chapter: complicating the experience of "collective biologies." In this book I have focused on one specific example of a collective biology: that of middle-class mestizo HIM participants incorporating local cultural common sense about the nature of Mexicanness into their hopes that individual health and gender behavior can enhance specific others' physical and social well-being. Like Catholicism and notions of machismo, this ideology of Mexican collectivity serves as an ambient cultural reference point. Yet focusing solely on how like-minded people draw on this pervasive cultural ideology risks painting that ideology as deterministic, universally accepted, or homogeneously experienced and used.

In practice, all participants drew on multiple worldviews to make sense of their lives. Some were widespread, such as the understandings of gender and personhood discussed as components of people's explanatory models of human papillomavirus (HPV) in chapter 2. Others related more directly to specific life experiences, such as the ethos of self-help shared by participants engaging in personal development or support groups. They also include a range of ideologies I have not yet discussed. For example, a few participants related medical research engagement to their activities selling health products through multilevel marketing companies. By promoting supplements, they sought to enhance others' health while also enhancing personal wealth in ways resonant with the entrepreneurial capitalist logics and middle-class aspirations promoted by their sales organizations (Cahn 2008).

In this chapter I focus on Cristianos' experiences as an example of how people drew on multiple worldviews to understand their lives—including medical research participation. I investigate how Cristiano participants drew on both secular and evangelical worldviews in their particular ways of incorporating HIM experiences into broader life efforts to enhance their own and others' well-being, in both the earthly and the spiritual realms. While Cristianismo is neither homogeneous nor deterministic of people's behavior, it offers a distinct understanding of the natures of personhood, embodied and spiritual interrelatedness, and collectivity that in some ways resonates with and in some ways diverges from the ideologies discussed previously.

Cristiano Takes on Health and Gender

Evangelical Christianities are faiths based in practice (Santos 2012). Since most Mexicans are born into Catholicism, Cristianos usually choose to convert and live out their faith through rituals, such as baptism, and daily-life changes that range from becoming vegetarian (in the case of Seventh-Day Adventists) to giving up extra- and premarital sexuality. The routine, banal activities of daily life thus become key sites in which Cristianos live out their faith. This understanding of piety as practice was emphasized in many of the discussions of theology in which I participated. For example, in a sermon I attended at a HIM participant's Adventist congregation, the pastor said that going to church was not sufficient. Instead, he said, piety required actively living church teachings through practices such as studying the Bible every day and avoiding alcohol. He explained that, to achieve salvation, people must both "evangelize" and "give testimony" (*testimonio*). The HIM participant's wife, Claudia, whispered to me that "evangelizing is telling people about Jesus Christ, and giving testimony is living a good life to model that."

Cristiano participants frequently voiced an understanding of piety as an ongoing, embodied practice that would create a godly internality. This echoed pervasive themes in Cristiano discourse, from sermons to small talk at church picnics and the articles in evangelical cooking magazines that Claudia lent me, regarding the need to focus on one's actions to live a godly life. For instance, this was highlighted in a vocal performance given at the Adventist church. Two young girls in ruffled party dresses, who were on tour from Mexico City to promote their Christian children's album, came to sing. One sang a song titled "Cuidadito" (roughly, "Carefully"), which listed the body practices through which children should live out their spiritual commitments in daily life. One verse was about washing your face before going to church; another was about how you have to be careful what your eyes see, what your hands touch, where your feet walk, what your mouth says, and what your brain thinks. "Cuidadito" was the refrain, reminding children to be ever-vigilant of the spiritual consequences of their everyday actions. This message highlighted both the need to embody church teachings in daily life and the focus of such messaging on health and hygiene, which ranged from hand washing for children to sexual continence for adults. This ideology enabled HIM participants and their partners to see sexual health research as a venue for living piously, especially by aligning their actions and bodies with the health, gender, and relationship ideals of their faiths.

Cristianismo offers an evangelical take on the kinds of gendered family relationships that have become ideal in mainstream Mexican culture. A source of appeal for growing Protestant faiths worldwide is their promotion of self-consciously modern forms of comportment, often framed as responses to societal dissolution. In the evangelical worldview, discipline and order in the individual and family are both signs of salvation and the method for achieving it. This includes modeling human submission to God via women's submission to a patriarchal order on Earth (Peterson et al. 2001). However, this vision of benevolent patriarchy includes dramatic reform of local masculinities to achieve a goal of religiously oriented companionate marriage, fidelity, and engaged fathering, as well as mothering (Berger and Hefner 2013; Garrard-Burnett and Stoll 1993; Van Klinken 2013).

This ideology can be attractive for both men and women. In sites where danger and economic privation make it difficult for men to meet provider ideals, Jose Leonardo Santos (2012: 37) notes, evangelical gender ideals enable men "to reclaim their masculinity by transforming it." Building on the anthropologist Elizabeth Brusco's (1993) foundational finding that conversion to evangelicism enabled Colombian men to engage in a "reformation of machismo," scholars in many world regions have identified such conversion as a way for men whose positions might be affected by cultural change, economic deprivation, or discrimination to reconfigure their ways of being men and thus achieve male privilege amid precarity (see, e.g., Dawley and Thornton 2018; Fesenmyer 2018; Heath 2003; Misra 2012; Van Klinken 2012). Conversion also offers emotional and social rewards for making such changes, from the promise of improved romantic relationships to the ability to engage emotionally with male peers while remaining seen as masculine (Dawley 2018; Flores 2014).

Women in Mexico and elsewhere are often drawn to evangelicism because of its potential to reconfigure masculinities that cause family suffering, making for still patriarchal but more companionate gender dynamics in the home (Douglas 2003; Everett and Ramirez 2015). Mirroring the masculine ideal of companionate responsibility, Cristianos critique machismo, seeking to direct men's activities toward salvation through the embodiment of benevolent patriarchy in which men lead through care rather than violent domination. Cristiano gender ideals thus echo but reframe broader cultural ideals of modern gender, calling for practices of masculinity and femininity that look similar to the mainstream versions in daily life but are set into an ideology not of egalitarianism but of benevolent earthly patriarchy mirroring a cosmically hierarchal relationship between God and humans. In Mexico, this concept can also resonate with broader class and racial ideologies—for example, enabling the enactment of modernity-identified practices such as companionate marriage through the daily-life performance of piety (Ramirez and Everett 2018).

Such evangelical takes on gender interrelate with ideals of health and self-care. Worldwide, evangelical churches often frame body practices such as regulating one's eating and abstaining from alcohol and drugs as ways to embody religious teachings and enact pious forms of personhood while also enhancing one's physical health (Hardin 2013; Magny 2009). Further, these practices are offered as ways to cope both spiritually and medically with the health problems wrought by preconversion behavior (Kelly-Hanku et al. 2014) and to offer behavioral protection against the health risks of impious sexuality and masculinity, such as HIV transmission (Smith 2004; Van Klinken 2013).

While faith healing is a key component of many evangelical faiths, churches—including those attended by participants in my study—often combine prayer with an emphasis on the use of biomedicine and the health-maintenance practices associated with modernity-oriented health cultures (Navarro and Leatham 2004). Like adherents to many world religions who incorporate high-tech medical intervention into religious practice (see, e.g., Inhorn 2003; Kahn 2000; Roberts 2006), Cristianos in the HIM study saw biomedical research as a productive site for living out their spirituality. Later I discuss how HIM participants and their partners incorporated this experience into broader efforts to embody religious ideals by aligning their bodies and behavior with church teachings regarding gender, marriage, family, and sexual and health practice.

Health Care as Piety

Cristiano participants saw God as the ultimate arbiter of health. In both congregations I visited, pastors appealed to Jesus as the "doctor of doctors," and parishioners told stories of miraculous healing caused by prayer in cases that biomedicine was powerless to cure. However, Cristiano participants and their churches also believed that preventative biomedical care and medically recommended lifestyle practices were important parts of a pious life. This practice of combining physical and spiritual interventions, including mixing systems based in science and faith, is extremely common throughout Mexico (Navarro-Hernández et al. 2018). People often move among very different modalities, such as biomedicine, *curanderismo*, and Eastern traditional medicine, as they search for relief and treatment that they can access and afford amid economic constraint (Napolitano 2002). Valentina Napolitano argues that choosing health interventions within this milieu also entails forging alignments with collective identities—such as membership in religious or political groups—and their politics. Writing about curanderismo and grassroots practice of *medicina popular* informed by Catholic liberation theology, Napolitano (2002: 127) notes that healing individual bodies explicitly entails treating ills in "the body of social and spiritual relations."

Cristiano HIM participants and their congregations engaged in such mixing by framing the use of biomedical interventions and lifestyle recommendations as a way not only to support, but also to actually embody the practice of piety that would ultimately provide healing. The hygiene exhortations of the "Cuidadito" song exemplify this. Notably, while the mixing of varied systems is common in Cuernavaca and elsewhere, Cristiano participants and their churches' health teachings focused on prayer and biomedicine. Their notable silence about traditional Mexican practices such as curanderismo likely reflects their broader rejection of folk Catholicism, efforts to assert mestizo and middle-class status, and alignment with their faiths' roots in North American culture.

This particular mixture of faith and science thus presented a modern way to perform piety. It meant that both prayer and adherence to biomedical recommendations were important ways that people lived out their faith. For example, Ana-María, a hairdresser and charismatic Christian, said that her church often held women's conferences: "They always bring doctors to teach us . . . , for example, about HPV or about the breasts or how to care for your nutrition." Based on what she learned through conferences and from health tips in church magazines, Ana-María implemented healthy behavior changes such as reducing her family's sugar intake. She saw this as a specifically religious duty, which had interlinked physical and spiritual benefits.

She also saw implementing biomedical lifestyle recommendations as her duty as a wife and mother, despite the church's similar health offerings for men. Laughingly acknowledging the tension between evangelical ideals of patriarchal yet care-oriented masculinities and the enduring feminization of care for family and health, she added that there are church health conferences "for men, too, except they don't go." Caring for her family's health was thus a multifaceted way for Ana-María to live out a feminine form of piety. It enabled her to treat her own and her loved ones' bodies as temples, which, in turn, involved doing the domestic work seen as befitting a good woman. This exemplifies how keeping one's family on a pious track becomes another form of women's domestic labor (Ramirez and Everett 2018). Further, it is one example of the globally common expectation that women should feed families in ways that simultaneously carry on valued traditions, support ideals of modernity, and mitigate "diseases of modernity" such as type 2 diabetes (Weaver 2018).

The belief that health was ultimately up to God but that one must still attend to it in daily-life behavior was characteristic of the practice orientation in Cuernavacan Cristianismo. For instance, behavior mattered more than words in Ana-María's church teachings. She noted, "Love isn't something you say. It's something you do. Love is action. So if they tell me there's something wrong, I change it." This change included altering health behavior that, with church guidance, she came to see as wrong. Ana-María saw her health and other lifestyle changes as ways to demonstrate her inner conversion, explaining that God "has changed my life totally and radically. It's that the values that I'd heard before, well, I've tried to put them into practice, to live them . . . , knowing God has helped me to be more aware [*consciente*] of myself, of my family, and of everyone around me." This emphasis on performing piety through care for oneself, one's family, and one's community extended even to the material world of the church: a sign in the restroom I visited at Ana-María's congregation said, "Show your love for the church by keeping the facilities clean." As in the "Cuidadito" song sung at a different congregation, this sign reminded participants that outward, embodied action both reflected and transformed one's spiritual interiority.

For Cristiano participants, health behavior served as one practice that united the spiritual and physical elements of faith. This was the case for Arturo and his wife, Ade, whose story opened this book. Ade had remained Catholic but was deeply interested in alternative healing and New Age spirituality, and she believed that physical sickness had a significant spiritual component. The couple believed that sinful lives caused emotional pain that, Ade noted, "we somaticize." She continued, "If people think that God is our creator and he has the power over everything. I think we can heal ourselves, we're interjecting that into our mind and the mind is driving the body." Arturo added, "Going to church cures your aches and pains and some diseases, with that [curative] health of the soul."

However, they viewed biomedical preventative care as an important supplement to spiritual hygiene. Ade lived this out in her work as a nurse, while Arturo believed that preventative health care was important for mitigating the physical ailments caused by people's poor preconversion life choices. He commented, "Ninety percent of us came to our religion. We weren't born into it, so we had unhealthy lifestyles first." He thus saw it as important to get checkups that would reveal health problems and engage in prevention. The HIM study served in part as a hygienic practice, akin to Adventist vegetarianism and sung reminders to carefully wash one's hands.

Like Arturo, other Cristiano participants often viewed the HIM study as an aid for redressing the health problems wrought by prior sinful behavior. The electrician Eusebio noted, "The Bible says that the body is a temple of God and that God's temple has to be clean." In keeping with that edict, he said, he had quit drinking, smoking, and womanizing when he converted. He viewed the HIM study's HPV testing as a way to monitor the lasting consequences of those actions. He remarked, "If I had obeyed God from the start, there wouldn't be any need for these talks with you, because I'd be physically healthy."

Some participants also thought that HIM involvement supported healthy lifestyles beyond the specific issue of sexual health. Ana-María understood the study experience of her husband, Juan, as a chance for them to review their health behavior as a couple. She told me that she always asked him about the health questionnaires Juan completed at each visit and said that discussing the topics made her think more about her own health. She called the questionnaires a "great help and blessing" "because they really touch on areas where often things are happening in our life but we don't notice," such as diet. She found such mindfulness of health behavior to be congruent with her church's teachings that "God's desire is that I be healthy." While Christ had healing powers, she said, fulfilling God's desire "depends on you" to live well.

Similarly, Claudia, a Seventh-Day Adventist, said that she enjoyed exercise but also was religiously required to be healthy because "we as Adventists have a certain diet" that is ideally vegetarian. She explained, "This isn't about prohibition but is something that you appreciate. It's for your own well-being. It liberates you from a lot of things." In our final interview, she discussed the need to care for one's health to maintain one's body in God's image. "If you eat a lot of grease, you get really fat," she said. "Physically, you look bad, because God didn't create human beings obese." She took the injunction to remake herself in God's image quite literally, seeking to engage in health behavior that would reshape her body—and, in the process, her soul—into what she saw as a godlier form.

Incorporating HPV Surveillance into Gendered Piety

Experiences with the HIM study thus became sites for living out ideal gender through religiously inspired health practice. Participants' congregations were explicitly patriarchal yet emphasized temperance and fidelity for men in ways that appealed to women. For example, Ana-María explained, "In my faith, God teaches us that men and women are equal in front of him. But in this world, there's a difference. The man is the head of the household, and we need to respect him. The woman also has a special place. Everyone has their place, even children. There's a specific order: God, Jesus, husband, wife, kids, family, others. This helps us have a good life."

This concept of gender complementarity and interdependence gave wives who met their expected familial duties the moral authority to call for men to change. Much of the religious discourse about piety, gender, and health involved calls on men to live out the anti-macho, care-oriented masculinities that were also being idealized as modern in the wider society. These kinds of masculinities were very visible in the Adventist and charismatic Christian churches I visited, where male preachers were the ultimate authorities but services featured many authoritative roles for women. There, fathers, as well as mothers, were intimately involved in childcare during the services. At one service, the lead pastor held his children while his wife preached as the man next to me lifted both of his young sons' hands in prayer, his sleeve shifting up to reveal the tattoo of a baby's footprint on his forearm.

Cristiano participants often discussed the changes men had made after converting. Ade, Arturo's wife, noted that, while Arturo had always been a good husband, conversion had "augmented" his positive traits of being "kind, calm, caring, attentive, a homebody" by also calming his tendencies to be "more controlling . . . , more demanding, quick to explode." Laughing, she noted that his change had led to a change in her own temperament: "Now I don't have anyone to yell at." Eusebio changed his behavior as a husband more dramatically after his conversion. When his wife, Elena, said that they used to have a "lack of respect," he interjected, "Now there's no cheating." She concluded that "his machismo" had made their marriage difficult but had improved since his conversion. Casting machismo as an innate but problematic trait that Cristianismo had helped him overcome, Eusebio explained, "As a man, a Mexican, [machismo] is something you have. But now I know that there are limits. I have the final word in the house. I'm the head of the household. If there's a problem, I'll work toward solving it. I'm not acting like a macho anymore." To take on the religiously requisite role of patriarch, he had needed to align his performance of masculinity with that promoted by the church.

Eusebio also incorporated his HIM study experiences into his adoption of this role. Incorporating the notion that his own bodily state would directly affect that of others, he found the knowledge that he could transmit HPV to be especially helpful for maintaining sexual continence. He explained how this knowledge had combined with his religious viewpoint to help him see that his past infidelity was harmful for everyone involved: "Now I know I'm a carrier. I think it wasn't fair that I put women at risk. I did it a lot, I suppose. I also feel like I brought the problem home." He also viewed this outcome as a direct consequence of failing to follow church teachings, noting,

> If I had listened to God that you have only one partner, I would not have given [my wife] the virus. . . . I lived badly, and this is the consequence. I have a virus. I'm a carrier. There's little chance that I'll get sick, but I can pass it on to my wife. I picked my wife [to marry] because I love her, but involuntarily I hurt her. The Bible shows us the path. The HPV reflects a bad decision.

Eusebio's emphasis on the negative health consequences that his infidelity had for his wife and his conceptualization of church teaching as a path to be actively followed reflect a combination of the societal ideal of male companionate responsibility with the practice orientation of Cristianismo. He noted that faith was not enough to make one a good man. Christians "aren't exempt from committing the same errors" as others, he said. Instead, he felt that his vulnerability called for constant deliberate action: "So we have to be constantly actualizing our practice [actualizándonos]."

Eusebio used medical research participation as one way of accomplishing those updates. He believed that the HIM study's sexual health surveillance, in addition to other sites of health behavior monitoring such as Alcoholics Anonymous, helped him to maintain his religiously mandated lifestyle changes. He said,

> I think that [the HIM study] was something that God prepared. . . . God gives the wound, and God heals the wound. Right? So I think

that's why I entered this study. . . . I didn't know that I had problems [with HPV], but I saw the opportunity and thought, well, I'll go. It's like when I went to Alcoholics Anonymous thirty-four years ago. They told me that they could help me, and I came to see that was true. . . . Now I'm here . . . to be under constant surveillance.

For him, the kind of surveillance that the HIM study and Alcoholics Anonymous offered were explicit supports for practicing the faithful, sober masculinity that the church promoted but that he felt his inherently macho nature made it difficult to enact.

For some couples, the HIM study experience became a site for negotiating maintenance of such masculine change. Ana-María said in our first interview that conversion had dramatically changed her marriage: "Before professing the faith, there were many problems at home. My husband drank: he was an alcoholic, and he liked the ladies. He was a womanizer. He even hit me a few times." She turned to religion for help coping with the death of one of her infants, and her husband eventually followed her lead. Both believed that his conversion had cured their surviving daughter's epilepsy, and Ana-María felt that it had radically improved their marriage.

However, over time her husband's observance wavered. In response, she invited him to our second interview and pointedly discussed his HPV test results in an attempt to remind him of the negative consequences of his preconversion behavior. In an ostensibly hypothetical statement about a man who "might have been unfaithful," she noted that HPV "has consequences, if not just the problem itself, it's that you bring it home to your partner. And the partner has a greater probability of contracting cancer . . . , if we're speaking in general terms, because the woman is more affected than the man." For Ana-María, the HIM study provided not only help for living a healthy and thus pious lifestyle, but also evidence of the physical wages of sin that, she hoped, would encourage her husband to stick to his postconversion habits.

In keeping with broader cultural trends, Cristiano discourses of gendered change emphasized the need to reject machismo. However, Christian women also incorporated HPV-related experiences and fears into their attempts to perform pious femininity. For instance, women as well as men saw preconversion sexual behavior that had led to HPV positivity as the wages of sin. Echoing Eusebio, Claudia said that church values such as fidelity help to prevent sexually transmitted infections (STIs), while the sin of fornication causes them. She explained that practices of sexual temperance "are values we've lost. That's why there are things like the virus [HPV]." She regretted that she had not always used condoms in prior relationships and saw her own HPV positivity as a direct consequence of both sexual sin and failure to care for her health. She had suffered a precancerous cervical lesion and worried about transmitting HPV to her husband. She thus appreciated that the HIM study provided him with HPV monitoring. She believed that medical surveillance was necessary for them as a couple to deal with the health consequences of her past bad behavior and that her religious faith, as well as the monogamy she practiced because of it, would ensure her future health and security. She said, "I asked God to help me, that the virus doesn't advance. But I know that actions have consequences. God will help me, but I have to look for how." The HIM study became one of many daily-life ways to help God keep her family healthy.

Another woman used knowledge of HPV risk gained through the HIM study to help herself conform to ideals of faithful femininity. Katia married her husband and converted to Mormonism to escape the oppressively religious grandmother who had raised her. While living with her grandmother, she said, "I was always stuck in church. . . . I didn't have male or female friends. I didn't go to parties. I didn't go anywhere. I didn't enjoy anything." Katia met her husband when she was fifteen and married him at nineteen without ever having been allowed to be alone with him. They had their first child when she was twenty, and she changed religions to escape the repression and "hypocrisy" of her grandmother's church.

While she said that she loved her husband and thought he was a caring partner and father, she discussed the temptation to cheat with another man during our second interview. She was deeply attracted to the man and resented that her husband had been able to sleep with another partner before they married but she had not. However, Katia thought that her desires were destructive and impious and told herself not to cheat. "I'd be a bad woman," she said. "I might feel bad as a woman. I'd feel bad with my family." She also saw the risk of contracting an STI that was highlighted by her HIM study involvement as a reason to avoid infidelity: "The other [reason] is the thought of the risk of some infection, of transmission." The specter of STI risk—and the social risk to her marriage posed by an STI diagnosis received in the planned women's study—helped her to conform to the ideal of faithful femininity. By the next year, Katia had refocused on her marriage, even asking her husband to accompany her to our interview to keep her company in transit. When we spoke privately, she said that she felt relieved of the stress of pondering infidelity.

Like Katia, participants often viewed pious gendered behavior as key for the companionate style of marriage that their churches, and the broader cultural discourse, framed as ideal. Choosing an observant Cristiano partner was a major theme in church teachings, as reported by participants and as I witnessed at church services. For instance, at the Adventist church, one of the pastors used women seeking husbands outside the faith as an example of the faithful being tempted by the devil. He warned the parishioners not to date outside the church, telling women not to care whether a man was handsome, but to focus on whether he was sober and faithful. He said that many women were lost to the church that way and did not "wake up" until they were abused by bad husbands or left as single mothers. In this vein, Claudia discussed her own earlier dating difficulties, saying that some men seemed to be Christian but were "two-faced," drinking and eating religiously prohibited meat when they were away from church peers. Cristiano participants overwhelmingly saw performing the masculinities and femininities that their churches required as requisite for ideally companionate marriages, as well as adherence to divine will that would provide earthly well-being and cosmic salvation.

In our interviews, participants often focused on how changes in their ways of being men and women facilitated companionate relations. For example, Arturo's wife, Ade, said that by enhancing his physical and emotional health, his conversion also improved their marriage. "We've learned that the important thing is your interiority and being well physically and emotionally," she said. "That's the key to deeper understanding, more spiritual [understanding]. Now we can talk through problems that arise. . . . We can analyze and solve them." Testing for STIs in the HIM study served to reveal bodily interiorities that directly indexed such spiritual interiorities. Engaging in such surveillance was one way that couples such as Eusebio and Elena and Ana-María and Juan emphasized that men's shifts away from macho behavior such as infidelity had improved their marital happiness.

Unlike older participants who had grown up at a time when men's infidelity was commonly viewed as a natural and normal behavior, young Cristiano participants viewed the HIM study not as an aid for men's change but as ongoing support for companionate, Christ-centered marriage. Luz, a Baptist lawyer, explained that her religion required men to care for their wives' health and well-being. Due to Mexican machismo, people often found men's infidelity acceptable, she said, but "in Cristianismo, it's not. They tell you to treat your wife like a fragile vase, made of glass or crystal, which you fill with your tenderness. She's not something foreign to you but part of you, part of your body." From this perspective, men's self-care, including through medical research participation, was actually a form of direct care for their wives as well as themselves. Emphasizing the centrality of the concept of couples biology to Cristiano ideology, Luz continued, "The Christian idea of marriage is that the two are one and what happens to one happens to the other." While participants in the broader anthropological study also often saw men's receipt of HPV testing as a way to care for wives' health, for Cristianos this also became a form of religious observance.

Luz and her husband, Jaime, a lab technician at the Instituto Mexicano del Seguro Social (IMSS) (see chapter 2), also incorporated joint HIM study attendance into their practices of marital togetherness. Both believed that Cristianismo had saved their natal families, causing what she called "an incredible transformation" in her parents' interactions and making his relatives shed their self-absorption so that they "finally took things as a family." They saw togetherness, in both spiritual and secular activities such as shared chores, as key to having the kind of intimate marriage the church promoted and that had transformed their relatives' relationships. So they reframed Jaime's individual HIM clinical visits as a couples event, attending them jointly and turning them into another site for performing togetherness. In fact, they compared the study visits to their weekly habit of cleaning the house together—something others (especially those in their social class, who usually relied on maids) saw as an unpleasant chore but that they viewed as a time for socializing and enacting familial care.

They also framed religiously requisite self-care as a collective act of companionacy. Both described themselves as people who, as Luz put it, "like to prevent" health problems and get routine medical testing. They incorporated this desire into their marital practice. Since Jaime worked at a medical lab, he sometimes gave Luz tests such as cholesterol screening. While Jaime had entered the HIM study several years before he met Luz, both thought that it helped their marriage. First, it demonstrated his concern for health maintenance. Second, it helped him nonjudgmentally to understand Luz's prior medical history, since she had had an HPV-related lesion removed before they met. Like Eusebio and Claudia, Luz and Jaime understood that infection as a remnant of Luz's preconversion past. Luz said that she had begun to drink and party in college, doing "things that can be damaging for you" before Christ "totally rescued my life." From that perspective, and using the information from the HIM study that HPV was common and usually not serious, they framed ongoing HPV surveillance as an opportunity for mutual support, togetherness, and eschewal of nonmodern and un-Christian masculinities that would lead a man to judge his wife for having premarital sex.

The HPV surveillance that the HIM study offered also enabled them to embrace the sex-positivity associated with this ideal of marriage. They believed the Baptist church provided a better guide to happy marital sexuality than Catholic cultural mores that promoted shame and silence. Jaime said the couple enjoyed sex "a thousand times more" than others because they understood that "God gave this to us to enjoy." Both also believed that the anti-macho mentality their church taught, which, Jaime explained, emphasized fidelity and "loving your partner in mind, body and soul," facilitated a good sex life. The ongoing HPV screening that Jaime received enabled both partners to feel relaxed about Luz's potential to transmit the virus, enabling them to enjoy sex without focusing on risks posed by their preconversion activities.

Spiritual and Earthly Motivations for Health Behavior

Cristiano participants thus understood HIM participation as one of many daily-life activities through which they could live out church-sanctioned forms of gender, health, and family. Involvement in medical research, like everything else, became a God-given opportunity to model the ideals of gender, health, and marital behavior promoted by their churches, which represented evangelically informed takes on pervasive local cultural ideologies. Like most study participants, Cristianos expected these efforts to enhance their embodied well-being and that of their loved ones. Yet while Cristiano participants incorporated their HIM experiences into earthly aspirations that looked broadly similar to those of the Catholic participants, the efforts were also profoundly influenced by—and expected, in turn, to influence—their existence in the spiritual realm.

Evangelical cosmology describes a world composed of three nested levels: the self, which is immersed in the society, which, in turn, is immersed in the cosmic level of God and the devil. In this worldview, individual actions have simultaneous and direct consequences for both one's society and the divine order (Santos 2012). Cristianos saw the cosmic level of scale as the most important one. However, they understood their fates in this realm to be contingent on their earthly efforts to embody God's model and to encourage others to do the same. This adds an extra dimension to the effort to model "living a good life" through which Claudia defined testimonio. As discussed in prior chapters, participants of all faiths discussed the importance of modeling desirable behavior to inspire behavioral change, and thus enhanced embodied well-being, in other members of their collective biologies. Yet the concept of modeling has more dimensions for Cristianos than for Catholic participants.

Most important for Cristianos is the individual effort to follow Jesus's model to embody spirituality in their daily-life behavior. Doing so has the primary benefit of strengthening the dyadic relationship between oneself and God in ways that will have positive spiritual consequences that will also be demonstrated through enhanced earthly well-being. Yet, as demonstrated by their efforts to promote godly living in family members, the study participants also hoped to have positive interactions with other people at the earthly societal level. In this way, modeling and promoting pious living would aid not only their own, but also others', salvation and terrestrial well-being. This logic of embodied interconnectedness is distinct from the common-sense local logic of Mexicanness as a collective biology. Yet these ideologies could comfortably exist alongside each other, since this mainstream cultural understanding of the earthly, societal level of scale did not conflict with evangelical theological understandings of the spiritual realm.

Cristiano participants thus drew on multiple ways of understanding their own actions as affecting the physical—and spiritual—fates of others as they engaged in health projects such as the HIM study. Such projects offered venues for enabling Cristianos to perform pious citizenship aimed at healing the earthly social bodies such as the Mexican populace and saving the souls that composed them. Arturo's story, which opened the book, illustrates how Cristiano participants incorporated HIM study participation into daily-life efforts toward these interlinked ends. His conversion was based in a response to endemic violence and reflected his desire to better live out the "modern" ideals of companionate marriage, male companionate responsibility, and engagement in preventative health care.

Arturo saw such efforts as not just individual practices of piety, but as elements of a collective congregational effort to heal the group's bodies and spirits. In his church, he noted, there are "alcoholics, drug addicts, and in the church we get healthy." This included both spiritual health and biomedical care. He reported frequently telling church friends that they should enroll in the HIM study to receive STI testing and mitigate the consequences of their "unhealthy lifestyles" prior to conversion. He also collaborated with "church sisters" to promote the use of state-sponsored health-screening programs. Together they promoted cervical cancer screening to parishioners but also lobbied politicians for more resources. He explained, "We went to see the municipal president to discuss [HPV] in women. Human papillomavirus has taken many women from our church, so we invite them to get testing, principally through [a federal agency that] . . . offers clinics for women and children." They thus sought to heal not only their own souls and bodies, but also those of others whom they could offer medical assistance.

Overall, Cristiano participants saw such medical offerings as venues that God presented them for living out his teachings and for encouraging others to do the same. As quoted earlier, Eusebio saw the study as "something that God prepared." Ana-María similarly saw state medical resources as divine opportunities to support the broader community's health, even as she cared for her own. She enrolled in a different IMSS HPV study that gave her a pap smear every six months, which she understood as a way "to help the community" by supporting scientific advances in addition to preventing harm to her health caused by her husband's preconversion infidelity. Evangelicism worldwide is often understood as part of a trend toward individualization, given these faiths' focus on personal behavior rather than work for structural change as a solution to earthly problems (see, e.g., Freeman 2014; Peterson et al. 2001). However, study participants fused this ethos with local cultural emphasis on interrelatedness in efforts to enhance both their own and others' embodied and spiritual well-being at the levels of couple, family, and society. They thus engaged in the broader cultural projects of cultivating a Mexican collective biology via specifically evangelical understandings of what collectivity might entail.

This intellectual linkage of personal and community benefit, on related spiritual and earthly levels, was not limited to the realm of health care. For instance, over the course of our interviews Claudia decided to return to school with the intention of becoming a nutritionist and helping her church community maintain their vegetarianism and health. After an aptitude test indicated she might be a good lawyer, her church community encouraged her to follow this more lucrative and high-profile path. She recalled, "I said I wanted to be a nutritionist to help the church, but they said, 'No, advance yourself.' Everyone was telling me I should be a lawyer." Her reticence related not only to the seeming loftiness of this goal but also to the difficulty of embodying godliness while practicing law during political crisis. "At first I didn't want to, because Mexico is very corrupt, so it's dangerous to me to be a lawyer here," she said. "As part of the church, I can't be corrupt. But God will help me." Claudia's plans and fears reflect her need to follow God's model, but to do so as a member of her church and of her broader society; she came to hope she could both better her own and her family's earthly life through her earnings and change a corrupt system from within through the fact of her difference from it.

Cristiano participants' understandings of all life opportunities—including medical research—as divinely ordained chances to aid themselves and others by engaging in testimonio and evangelism were demonstrated in their desire for the HIM staff to know that God had planned and sanctioned their work. For instance, Elena, Eusebio's wife, praised the study for providing men's HPV testing. When I asked whether there was anything she would change, she said that the HIM study and research science in general should be more explicit about attributing their findings to God. She explained, "God says that he gave science to man, but sometimes man decides that he discovered it and doesn't always give the honor to God."

Participants seemed to see my anthropological research in this way, as well. For participants such as Ana-María, our interviews became a discursive space for promoting the faith—in some cases, encouraging one's spouse to remain observant, and in others, proselytizing to me. Ana-María came to see her participation in my study as part of a divine plan for her to convert me, telling me that we had met and I had attended her church "for a reason." Similarly, Elena used the final moments of our last interview to proselytize to me. "I don't think this was just coincidence," she said about her own and Eusebio's recruitment to HIM and my anthropological research. "This is so that you can learn and know that there is a God." As we hugged after our final interview, she whispered, "Read the Bible."

Prayer's Power for Individuals and Collectives

Beyond the fact that they understood the spiritual level of scale to be a primary motivator of their own health behavior and their promotion of that behavior to others, Cristianos understood collectivity in an additional way. What people called the "church family" was a collective in some ways akin to the collective biologies of the couple, family, and Mexican society discussed in prior chapters. Just as it offers an evangelical revision of locally mainstream gender and health ideals, Cristianismo offers an ideology of individuals as parts of a broader whole that is distinct from, yet resonates with, the idea of Mexicans as parts of a mestizo biosocial body.

Social scientists have long understood group worship as a site for cultivating intensely embodied experiences of interconnectedness (Durkheim [1912] 2008; Turner 2012; Turner 1969). This was quite apparent in the congregations I visited. For instance, at a charismatic Christian megachurch, prayers and high-energy interludes of live Christian rock music were accompanied by a dance team of more than one hundred children in collective motion. Wearing matching tunics, they filled the church aisles and risers, waving flags in rhythmic choreography. One Sunday, the boys each held two blue flags while the girls held sparkling hula hoops, which they waved, tossed, and spun as the band reached a crescendo. Their performance made visible the physical size and unity of the church family and highlighted the shared nature of their pious practice through the visual metaphor of shared movement. Sermons then put this emphasis on the congregation as a spiritual collective into narrative form—for example, by emphasizing that while one's ills would be healed by God, one should seek that divine healing relationship through interpersonal and shared immersion in the daily life and practice of the church community.

Yet beyond the experiential power of community, Cristiano worship explicitly promoted the idea that the individuals in the congregation, and especially the congregation as an aggregate of these individuals, had a specific spiritual power to effect embodied change in others within the earthly realm. Beyond influencing others through modeling or evangelizing, Cristianos were told to use their embodied power of prayer to directly affect others' health and well-being. The simultaneously spiritual and corporeal nature of such power was demonstrated to me the first time I attended Ana-María's church. After asking me about my religious background, she and her sister explained that, while they were "adopted" into Jesus's family, I as a Jew was his direct relative. They understood this biological kinship with Jesus to mean that I had inherited spiritual powers. After praying they asked me to touch and bless them. When I did, Ana-María's sister stiffened as if struck by a lightning bolt and fell straight backward on the concrete floor, sobbing in tongues. Ana-María explained, "This must look strange to you, but she's got the spirit. You've given her a great blessing. You are very special." The power that they believed me to be invested with came from two sources: my membership in Jesus's literal family body and the power of an individual's prayer to create physically embodied spiritual response in others. In a religious take consonant with the broader cultural ideas that couples, family, and social bodies were physically as well as socially interrelated, Cristianos saw spirituality as a concrete force that could directly affect the bodies of those related through family, biological, social, and spiritual relationships.

This notion underlay the idea that individuals' prayers could have direct spiritual and health consequences for others navigating the local violence crisis. For example, at Ana-María's church pastors led prayers asking God to "keep the kidnappers out of our houses, out of our church," thus seeking to intervene in the actions of those kidnappers through God as a conduit. Individual parishioners were also told that they were responsible for the collective well-being of their society through personal, pious action. For instance, in one sermon a pastor noted that, since "the world is going to hell," the faithful should evangelize as much as possible, because if they did not, they, like Oskar Schindler, would die wishing they had saved "just one more." The pastor asked how they would feel if they got to heaven and their spouse, kids, coworkers, or classmates were not there. Reinforcing the idea that Cristianos were responsible for the salvation of others, he suggested sending Facebook messages to Mexican celebrities in the hope that their high-profile conversions would serve as models to others throughout the nation. In this ideology, the world is doomed, and individual action is key for one's spiritual well-being. In turn, these individual acts of piety have direct consequences for both the earthly and eternal well-being of others. Praying for others, converting them, and modeling pious behavior for them becomes a direct way to influence their health and safety, in this world and the next.

In addition to promoting the use of individual prayer to affect other individuals, these congregations emphasized the ways that their collective action could reshape their worldly context. For instance, a pastor at Ana-María's church said, "We need to pray to bring God to Cuernavaca," and "Having a loud voice in praise [can turn things around]." He asked the congregation to reflect on recent murder victims who had died without knowing Jesus and to pray for everyone, including those who commit violence, assaults, kidnappings, and murders. He next told us to think of our neighborhoods and pray for everyone in them. Splitting the massive auditorium into two halves, he asked one side to pray for the governor and the other to pray for the municipal president. Finally, he led us in a more formal prayer, asking these politicians to come to "the light of Christ." The implication of this sermon was that the congregation's collective prayer could have two kinds of direct, embodied effects on others that could ameliorate the local violence. Praying and living piously could save the souls of criminals, who would then stop harming others, and collective prayer could exert a direct force on politicians, whose own salvation would model piety for others and lead to better governance that could physically protect local citizens in their earthly lives.

This aim of helping others spiritually and physically through the power of prayer was distinct from the idea of modeling healthy behavior for others in the mestizo collective biology. Prayers were expected to reach God, who would then effect change in others. This was a different way of fomenting change through interrelatedness from the efforts discussed in prior chapters. Similarly, Cristianos' efforts to perform testimonio by modeling pious practice were first and foremost about following Jesus's model in ways that would then serve as a model for others in the earthly realm.

Combining Ideologies

Like other participants, Cristianos used their HIM experiences as venues for embodying and modeling their takes on local ideals of gender, marriage, and political commitment. Yet they understood medical research participation primarily through an evangelical worldview. Their narratives thus emphasized the spiritual level of scale and the ways that earthly pursuits, including the HIM study, would affect their own and others' fates within it. Nevertheless, their understandings of events in the terrestrial realm also appeared to be influenced by the local cultural ideologies of collectivity discussed earlier. While evangelical faiths focus on individual behavior as the path to salvation, participants' understandings of themselves as components of nonindividual bodies were also central to the ways in which they performed prayer, testimonio, and evangelism—and thus sought to save their own and others' souls.

For the Cristianos in this study, the belief that one's individual actions have direct consequences for broader social bodies appeared to come from dual sources, promoted by both the ideology of mestizaje and by their Christian theology. Both ideological realms place similar emphasis on achieving good personhood by living out ideal forms of gender, marriage, and self-care. Yet they look to different ends, in the service of different collectives; mainstream cultural discourses of modernity seek to heal the mestizo social body, while Cristiano ideology focuses on divine salvation. As the HIM participants discussed earlier understand their personal body practices to affect others in a racially interrelated body, Cristiano participants additionally saw acts such as medical research participation as impacting the broader wholes of the congregation and the cosmic world subsuming the mortal level of existence.

Cristiano participants drew on these multiple ideologies to guide their daily-life actions at the individual, couple, and societal levels of scale discussed in the prior chapters. For instance, they incorporated their medical research experiences into individually oriented efforts to perform and maintain church-sanctioned behavior. Repeated HPV testing offered participants incentives to continue espousing anti-macho masculinities, family-oriented femininities, and companionate relationships by highlighting the consequences of sexuality not sanctioned by the church. Participants simultaneously saw the testing as a form of preventative health care that could help them perform religiously required care for themselves and their romantic partners while also helping them to cope medically with the consequences of their preconversion behavior.

In their discussions of couples-level well-being, Cristianos' hopes for HIM participation and other health behavior represented an evangelical take on the Mexican cultural notion that individuals are inherently interrelated through shared biology and behavioral tradition. Through modeling piety and evangelizing about faith in interview encounters with their spouses and researchers like me, they hoped to keep their spouses faithful to church teachings. Like Catholic participants, they understood the couple's body as a biologically and socially intertwined unit in which one person's sexual hygiene and health behavior directly affected the other's health. Yet this relationship represented the embodiment of an even more important spiritual component. They understood care for the couple's body as a practice of piety and as a way to be a caring spouse—as Jaime put it, loving one's partner in "soul" as well as "mind" and "body."

Although evangelical faiths worldwide cast "worldly" life as a distraction from the key business of salvation to be lived out individually and within the family, Cristianos also hoped to effect change in the ailing Mexican social body through their pious action. At the level of the social body, doing testimonio by living well through activities such as medical research participation represented a way to save others in the process of saving oneself. Participants hoped not only to influence loved ones, but also to combat violent societal dissolution through modeling, prayer, and evangelization that would convert the criminals and politicians responsible for harm.

Such hopes for effecting societal change by relating in both earthly and spiritual ways with others reflected a specifically Cuernavacan Cristiano understanding of collectivity or interrelatedness. Beyond the prevailing cultural ideology of people as parts of a broader Mexican whole, Cristianos saw shared human frailty and fallibility as the biosocial nature that bound people together. While all participants often said, "As Mexicans, we . . . ," Cristianos similarly discussed shared human nature, as in Ade's statement, "We're human beings, and we're weak, and we fall into temptation." Participants fused such ideas of shared human vulnerability to sin with the notion that people could change their behavior to overcome innately Mexican failings of machismo and lack of health culture—and, in the process, encourage others to do the same. Jaime explained that Cristianismo alters one "psychologically, socially, and culturally, taking into account that you struggle against what your culture is, and all it involves. . . . You go against the current to demonstrate that a deity has a plan for your life." Through wide-ranging activities, including medical research participation, they opposed cultural currents of machismo and lack of a culture of prevention in ways that reflected a fusion of cultural tropes of collectivity with evangelical cosmology.

For these additional reasons, Cristiano participants shared the opinion voiced by many other participants that they were uniquely well positioned to heal the ailing social body through their own actions. While they emphasized individual behavior and cast earthly concerns as potentially diabolical distractions from the pious living that would grant eternal salvation, they nevertheless directed this focus on individual salvation toward shoring up state systems, from politics to health care. Just as HIM participants and their partners in general saw themselves as a middle-class vanguard who could lead the Mexican social body forward, Cristianos saw themselves as a spiritual vanguard who could promote salvation—and its physical, psychological, and spiritual benefits. Focusing on piety as the primary qualifier for this leadership, rather than class status or educational attainment, made the privilege available to the socioeconomically diverse group of Cristiano participants, who ranged from wealthy professionals to economically precarious laborers.

In sum, Cristianos' narratives show how people might combine varied ideologies to make sense of a particular life experience. These participants drew on multiple, sometimes overlapping and sometimes diverging, culturally intelligible ways of understanding the consequences that research involvement could have for themselves and others. Despite foci on the individual in both medical research design and evangelical cosmology, they fused local understandings of collectivity into their hopes for effect in the earthly realm, which they, in turn, understood as part of a broader spiritual world and path.

Participants' hopes that activities such as HIM participation could heal biosocial-spiritual collectives, mediated by the ideologies discussed here, demonstrate the need to understand medical research participation at multiple levels of scale. The spiritual realm was omnipresent in these participants' explanations of even their most mundane behavior and experiences. For them, engagement with medical research thus necessarily entailed a spiritual dimension. While study researchers, including myself, understood themselves to be engaged in a secular project of investigation, Cristiano participants characterized research involvement as a divinely ordained opportunity for testimonio and evangelism. As I discuss in the next chapter, examples such as this highlight the need to look beyond individual bodies to fully understand the consequences of activities such as health research, even in the presence of individualizing discourses.

SEVEN

FROM "HUMAN SUBJECTS" TO
"COLLECTIVE BIOLOGIES"

This book opened with the story of Arturo, whose path to medical research participation began in the trunk of his stolen taxicab rather than a clinic. Arturo's choice to start telling me the story of his medical research participation by describing his carjacking shows how his enrollment in the Human Papillomavirus Infection in Men (HIM) study was about much more than monitoring his individual biology. Arturo eventually joined the HIM study as just one of many efforts to live out the new ways of being a husband and father that he promised God he would make if he survived his ordeal. He made meaning of his experience of violence by focusing on his relationships, striving to enhance the health and well-being of his couple's, family's, congregation's, and society's bodies through pious and progressive action. His HIM participation became a tool for engaging in these broader projects of collective well-being after directly suffering from the effects of its breakdown.

My goal in this book has been to honor the efforts of participants such as Arturo by shedding light on the collectively oriented aspects of ostensibly individually focused and clinically bounded medical research. I have analyzed Arturo's and other HIM participants' experiences of being "human subjects" of medical research as they themselves experienced them: as aspects of broader, collaborative efforts to be good and healthy partners and citizens as they cared for others amid changing ideals of masculinity, marriage and family, and a narcoviolence crisis fueled by government corruption. This study shows one way that people imagined and promoted collective well-being as they saw the tenuous gains of modernity and government systems of care crumble around them. It reveals one case of a broader phenomenon that, as I discuss later in this chapter, has major consequences for public health and bioscientific practice.

To understand research participation in this way I have analyzed interviews with couples based in, but looking outward from, the clinic. I have followed the links they made between their shared experiences of men's research involvement to the daily life sites and the romantic, familial, civic, and spiritual relationships that motivated their participation and that they hoped it would benefit. To analyze their experiences, I have built on scholarship revealing the importance of structural and cultural forces and inequalities as key shapers of global medical research and its consequences (see, e.g., Abadie 2010; Epstein 2008a; Fisher 2008; Petryna 2009).

This work and my own applies the fundamental anthropological insight that gender, race and other ideas of what makes someone a person emerge from our daily-life interactions with our cultural, interpersonal, and material environments—including medical research studies. The social-science literature on people's experiences of medical research uses that approach to identify how the enshrinement of individualistic Euro-American understandings of personhood, which frame research participation as an altruistic act divorced from daily life needs or context, has obscured consequences of medical research that occur beyond the level of individual participants and their biology or clinical experience (see, e.g., Montoya 2011; Morris and Bàlmer 2006; Sariola and Simpson 2011; Shaw 2017; Towghi and Vora 2014). Those findings and mine contribute to a reframing of health behavior as a potentially outward- as well as inward-looking practice through which people might seek to contribute to societal-level changes, as well as monitor and express the embodied effects of their social and structural contexts (cf. Broholm-Jørgensen et al. 2019). As I discuss later, my findings about the concrete biosocial effect of men's HIM participation on broader collective and context-specific biologies demonstrate how integrating social-science analysis into medical research from the design stage onward could help it to assess the biological changes it seeks to study more accurately, faithfully, and fully.

In this book, I have sought to meet the calls emerging from social-science literature on clinical trial participation to understand how relationships at multiple "levels of scale" shape the nonindividual effects of medical research participation (Geissler 2011; Molyneux and Geissler 2008; Whyte 2011). This multiscalar approach has been fundamental to my project from data collection onward. For instance, taking couples rather than individuals as my fundamental unit of analysis centered participants' hopes for HIM involvement not in the often individualistic frameworks of clinical bioethics but, instead, in their own relational experiences of daily-life decision making (Al-Mohammad 2012; Kingori 2013). I traced these hoped-for consequences out from the couple to broader levels of scale by attending to participants' and their partners' stated hopes of enhancing the well-being of a series of nested biosocial groups to which they felt they belonged. Investigating relationships across these levels of scale in this setting has enabled me to theorize the relationships between influential cultural logics, such as those regarding gender, race, and modernity, and people's experiences of medical research participation.

Focusing on a longitudinal, observational medical study, rather than a clinical trial, also helped me to highlight the relational aspects of research participation across both relational and temporal scales. This look at people's experiences over time adds productive complexity to the visual metaphor of nested levels of scale that I have used throughout the book. I have used the figure of concentric levels of experience to conceptualize how people's individual bodily experiences are contextualized in the experiences of their dyadic romantic relationships, which, in turn, are set within their families, and those are set within their broader society. Yet these interrelationships are not nested and bounded in the static way suggested by the image of a set of Russian dolls. Instead, participants' discussions of change over time show that all of these levels are porous and shifting. Romantic relationships begin and end and are influenced by partners' past romances. Family structures change as partners blend children from prior relationships and children grow up. Society on the broadest level is dramatically changed by forces such as economic crisis and the rise of violence. People also experience these changing and interrelated levels of scale by applying diverse and changing ideologies, as demonstrated by those participants who combine the logics most prevalent among study participants with evangelical theology in chapter 6. My goal here is to discuss the ways that ongoing, embodied changes on all of these levels interrelate in ways that relate to people's daily-life experiences, including medical research participation.

This approach also broadens our understanding of the consequences of longitudinal medical research. This form of health research has rarely been studied by social scientists. Yet the long-term medical surveillance it involves can both influence participants' life experiences over the long term and offer a forum for them to live out ongoing and collaborative projects of personhood. As I discuss later in this chapter, when I provide suggestions for incorporating the study of collective biologies in health research and similar pursuits, these findings can help us to understand the nonindividual, biosocial ramifications of the ever-increasing forms of health surveillance and experimental treatment in use worldwide (e.g., Armstrong 1995; Hughes et al. 2018).

The Findings

I have based my analysis of the HIM study's collective consequences on the areas of life most significant, changing, and fraught for the middle-class, heterosexual Cuernavacan participants. My focus on this group broadens the scope of social-science knowledge about the consequences of medical research participation, since investigations of this topic have focused primarily on socially and economically marginalized populations seeking care and resources from globalized medical research (e.g., Elliott and Abadie 2008; Geissler and Molyneux 2011; Petryna 2009).

Studying Mexican HIM participants' experiences reveals how people can incorporate health research participation into broader—specifically, middle-class—modernity projects. Involvement in the HIM study was one of many ways that participants sought to maintain social status and stability by providing an arena for living out self-consciously modern forms of gender, family, and citizenship, despite destabilizing violence and economic crises. Enrollment in the study also enabled participants to see themselves as leading the Mexican populace forward by example in a cultural context in which national narratives of Mexicanness have cast individual behavior as the engine of population-level modernization via the ongoing process of mestizaje. Such narratives have focused on families as key sites for this modeling (see, e.g., Stern 1999). Study participants' experiences, too, reveal how heterosexual couples might understand themselves as building blocks of their broader society, tasked with advancing society by rearing more modern children. These couples' experiences thus provide one of many global examples of middle classes driving cultural quests for modernity by using the tools of global capitalism, even as it threatens their precarious gains (Freeman 2014; Inhorn 2012; Sumich 2016).

The participants' stories also demonstrate how this global trend plays out in a particular kind of context: a site where people see relationality rather than individualism as most fundamental to being a person, modern or otherwise. This analysis of HIM participants' and their partners' experiences thus shows how they expected medical research participation to do real physical good for the nonindividual bodies to which they belonged. In the Cuernavacan context, this included supporting medical advancement and living out and modeling ideals of gender and race. These historically have been promoted as key ways of living out "healthy" and "modern" Mexican personhood and appeared so today to the middle-class participants coping with government unreliability and violent crisis that threatened the nation's progress toward modernity.

I have introduced the concept of collective biologies to discuss such nonindividual understandings of biology and society. Collective biologies are biosocial groups whose interrelated behaviors and bodies can be influenced by the actions of those who form parts of these larger wholes. It is quite obvious to say that people's social and physical states are interrelated with those of other people, beings, and things in their environment. The concept of collective biologies is thus intended to demarcate one particular kind of interrelatedness and make it possible to study. This is the biosocial interrelatedness lived out by those who experience belonging in a specific, culturally defined collective. For HIM participants, such collectives included "Mexicans" and "our family." This means not that national populaces and families everywhere should be analyzed as collective biologies, but that in this ethnographic context, people believed that these entities were discrete, bounded units composed of individuals whose experiences profoundly influenced the embodied well-being of the unit as a whole, and thus of the other people belonging to it. While I have employed this concept to analyze HIM participation in Mexico, later in this chapter I discuss how it could be used to understand the nonindividual consequences of medical research and health surveillance in other settings where ideologies of collective biology are relevant.

In this Mexican setting, I have used this analytic approach to reveal how middle-class, heterosexual Cuernavacans are using ostensibly individualistic medical research to enhance collective well-being amid social change and violent crisis. Their efforts focused on a series of nested, biosocial bodies that were simultaneously physical and symbolic. In chapter 2 I investigated the smallest of these levels of scale, discussing men's narratives of gendered selfhood in relationship to HIM experience. I discussed their efforts to incorporate medical research involvement into sometimes long-standing and sometimes new performances of companionate responsibility, done in relationship to an enduring ideology of Mexican machismo as problematic yet intrinsic to mestizo biology and culture. By examining how men experienced themselves as men, both in relationship to membership in this abstract group of "Mexican men" and in their lived relationships with wives and others, the chapter also shows the "individual" level of gendered selfhood to be fundamentally relational in context-specific ways.

Chapter 3 focused on the level of couples biologies. Beyond simply seeing a person who has tested positive for the human papillomavirus (HPV) as having the capacity to infect a spouse through sexual contact, partners understood their physiologies as collective rather than individual in important ways. They understood shared bodily states, including but not limited to viral transmission, to be fundamentally influenced by both partners' actions, including collaboration to perform particular kinds of love, marriage, family, and health behavior. They also saw these biologies, as well as who counted as a *portador/a* (carrier), as profoundly influenced by performances of gender that they understood as also intimately related to their shared biosocial inheritance as Mexicans. In this context, the social consequences of HPV positivity depended on the happiness of people's marriages, especially male partners' ability to live up to the ideal of faithful, companionate responsibility. The chapter thus demonstrates how the ideologies of gender and Mexicanness participants articulated in chapter 2 shaped their explanatory models of HPV, as well as their accounts of its social risk.

Chapter 4 discusses spouses' incorporation of men's HIM enrollment into broader efforts to be good parents and raise modern companionate families. Participants understood medical research participation to provide family-level benefits, such as ensuring that parents would be healthy enough to support their children and enabling them to teach self-consciously modern and, they hoped, health-promoting gender and marital practices by example. I also discuss how parents' hopes for creating progressive families relied on contrasting themselves with imagined, less modern others in ways that reified ideas of machismo as inherently Mexican, as well as the class and racial hierarchies central to Mexican inequalities.

Chapter 5 focuses on people's hopes for aiding the Mexican social body by embodying change within it. The chapter shows how, given that goal, ostensibly individual medical research participation became a form of citizenship and civic activism. Participants sought to model and promote a "culture of prevention" that, participants feared, Mexicans as a biosocial group were innately predisposed to lack. These health-promoting actions also enabled them, as exemplary citizens participating in the kind of modern health behavior that the government had long promoted, to make calls on the Mexican government for promised but unreliably delivered security and care. The chapter shows how an ideology of collective biology enabled participants and their partners to use their own health and civic behavior in efforts to change the fate of the Mexican populace. Acting as citizens in a racial whole that they saw as affected by, but not identical to, the Mexican state, and guided by the ideology of health through modernity that the state had long promoted, participants used HIM involvement as one of many daily-life practices of citizenship through which they sought to promote population well-being, despite state failings.

Chapter 6 shifted the focus to Cristiano participants, who incorporated spiritual ideas of relatedness into their medical research experiences in addition to the ideologies discussed earlier. I discussed how they used HIM participation as one of many ways to help meet the goals of *testimonio* (pious living)—by acting healthfully, creating domestic and sexual harmony, and combating societal dissolution in the specific ways promoted by their churches. I used their emphasis on religion as an example of the broader truth that all participants drew on multiple ideologies to develop goals and make sense of their actions and experiences, including those related to the HIM study. Thus, chapter 6 contextualizes the book's primary focus on participants' use of a local ideology of collective biology within the more complex ideological context of daily life. In so doing, it also complicates the model of nested levels of scale I use to discuss interactions between individuals and collective biologies. It shows how the spiritual realm can both represent a broader level of scale enfolding the concentric levels of the couple, family, and Mexican society and cross-cut and complicate lived experience on those levels by serving as one of many ideologies on which people might draw to guide that experience. Since religious belonging is a key way that many people worldwide understand themselves and their membership in varied collectives (see, e.g., Castor 2017), I also hope that this analysis demonstrates the utility of the concept of collective biologies for understanding the interrelated social, physical, and spiritual experiences of membership in a religious collective.

I focus on the HIM study as a site for articulating understandings of collective biology to challenge the assumption within bioethics from the global North that people participate in studies due to a generalized sense of altruism. In this case, study participants hoped to get specific benefits from HIM participation, for themselves and for others, which evolved in response to their changing lives over the course of the study. These benefits included medical testing for participants and their partners, aiding in the advancement of medicine that would help the Mexican social body, supporting the local research infrastructure, and the opportunity to model positive health and gender behavior.

These hopes were mediated by a range of locally culturally intelligible ideologies, from gender norms to evangelical Christianities. Here I have focused on how they were significantly influenced by a specific idea of collective biology related to understandings of modern Mexicanness, including the raced and gendered components of that ideology. This focus reflects my goals of challenging the universality of expectations for research participant behavior based in Anglo-American ideas of individualistic personhood and of providing a clear analytic for conceptualizing people's hopes of influencing others with whom they see themselves as related in directly physical, as well as social, ways. The analysis here demonstrates that ideologies of biocultural collectivity were central to people's efforts to derive meaning and benefit from HIM involvement while the logics that underlay those ideologies, such as local ideas of race and gender, were sometimes explicit and sometimes coded or implicit in their narratives.

The book also shows how medical research can be a site for pursuing broader life goals and projects. The HIM study was generally a peripheral rather than a central aspect of people's daily lives, yet it served—like other life experiences—as one of many venues through which participants sought to care for their own and their loved ones' health, live out desired forms of personhood, and promote these forms of personhood to others. I focus on their medical research experiences as the center point for understanding these broader projects because this realm of experience has too often been conceptualized within social science and public health as separate from and unrelated to people's overarching life goals and webs of interpersonal interaction. As HIM participants' narratives demonstrate, understanding that relatedness is necessary for identifying the full range of embodied consequences that medical research participation can have.

Finally, it is important to note that participation in the HIM study did not always serve as a source of support for such endeavors. As demonstrated by the hurt and anger voiced by many people in chapter 3, participants often received unanticipated positive diagnoses that created problems in their relationships. They also voiced frustration at the limits of the study, which ranged from the nonmaterialization of a hoped-for study of female partners to Cristianos' complaint that study staff failed to recognize the hand God played in their work. These limitations were very apparent in the case of Abel and Blanca (see chapter 4). Abel tried and failed to use his HPV test results—along with other forms of evidence, such as his efforts to work, despite disability—to convince Blanca of his fidelity and worthiness as a husband. She remained unconvinced of his claims, and of the utility of medical research participation, staying with her husband and attending our interviews based on her sense of duty alone. Such experiences—or simply less enthusiasm for the HIM project—were likely more common among those not recruited for my study. Nevertheless, it is notable that so many participants did understand themselves to have incorporated an ostensibly individual experience of health surveillance into broader life efforts to help themselves and others.

IMPLICATIONS FOR UNDERSTANDING COLLECTIVITY AMID PRESSURES TO LIVE INDIVIDUALLY

These specific findings on people's ideas of themselves as components of broader collective biologies based on local ideologies of race, kinship and religion demonstrate both the commonness and the context-specificity of nonindividual understandings of biology. The Cuernavacan HIM participants prided themselves on modeling "modern" health and gender practices but did not adopt the individualistic focus built into globalized medical research. Instead, they drew on ideas of personhood as fundamentally relational, drawing implicitly on the cultural trope of Mexicans as interrelated by an ongoing process of modernizing away from indigeneity via mestizaje, to use medical research as one of many ways to "live for" others. This approach links people such as Marta and Antonio (the "mother hen" parents introduced in chapter 4) with people who seek to live for others in other difficult times and places (see, e.g., Al-Mohammad 2010). People such as the driver Javier understood themselves primarily as "grains of sand" on a larger biosocial beach rather than as isolated individuals. Here I have used the concept of collective biology to understand how such understandings of themselves as parts of broader biosocial wholes influenced participants and partners' actions. I have also used it to make visible the social and physical health consequences of men's research participation not captured in official HIM study findings, including its effects on other members of broader biosocial bodies.

The analysis in this book models a way to understand how people employ collectivist ideas of personhood amid increasing neoliberalism. In neoliberal ideology, discussed in chapter 5, people are increasingly encouraged to care for themselves in individualistic ways rather than to engage with and rely on community- or national-level support systems, facilitating those systems' privatization (Saad-Filho and Johnston 2005). This worldview is influencing policies and daily lives worldwide, but people complexly incorporate it into, rather than substitute it for, preexisting ideologies such as collectivist ideas of personhood (Kingfisher and Maskovsky 2008; Ong 2006). As Susanna Trnka and Catherine Trundle (2014) argue, the increasing pressure to take responsibility for monitoring and combating individual risks does not lead only to individualizing ideas about health and care. Instead, people idealize and seek to perform varied kinds of responsibility. These can include mutual forms of care based on ideologies of interrelatedness and collective calls on states and institutions to live up to social contracts.

Social scientists have been documenting the ways that people create new social groups to meet health, resource, and emotional needs related to shared biological experiences. By forming new collectives, people can call on governmental resources through the act of demonstrating belonging (Petryna 2003; Rabinow 1999; Rose and Novas 2005). They can also seek resources from nonstate institutions and collectives when governments fail to provide care. P. Wenzel Geissler (2015: 35) notes that investigating the context-specific ways that people come together to claim resources can help us to understand both the "unpredictable processes of collectivization and consciousness" that can arise from shared experiences of surveillance and emerging forms of "civic commitment" that seek communal care despite unreliable governments. This book has shown how HIM participants and their partners sought to accomplish this in the service of preexisting collectives by serving as model users to call for promised federal health care while seeking to support a mestizo social body affected by, but not identical to, the Mexican state.

Researchers have identified other cases in which Mexican patients and health professionals have infused individually focused biomedicine with local emphasis on relatedness as fundamental to personhood. Clinicians report seeking "Mexican model[s]" of mental health treatment that take interconnected kin or social groups rather than individuals as primary (Lester 2007: 377). This is the case in the "family constellations therapy" being practiced in Oaxaca State, where family is the primary unit of intervention and members are seen as explicitly relationally embodied (Duncan 2017). It has also been documented in psychiatric treatment in the city of Puebla, where physicians focus not only on individual patients but also on the kin networks that will provide care and help prevent relapse as primary to treatment of patients' mental health issues (Hale 2017).

Such collectively oriented responses to individualizing phenomena are also visible in Mexican people's responses to state failures to provide promised care. Despite its explicit goal of providing care for the social body, the postrevolutionary welfare state has not lived up to its promises and has engaged in massive privatization (MacLeod 2004). Yet Mexican citizens continue to decry this approach (see, e.g., Vergara 2016) amid powerful protests against government corruption and collusion in narcoviolence that have drawn on collectivist ideologies (Adler 2012). Engagement in medical research by HIM participants for collective good, including as a way to model modern use of government health-care resources to justify calls for more support, demonstrates a less visible form of such protest. Yet this is one of a range of collectivist responses to the failures of a corrupt state cutting its promised, shared safety net.

In addition to calling on the government to enhance support, Mexicans in some cases have created alternative collectives centered on varied forms of relatedness. These include anticapitalist organizing around Indigenous identity, the formation of "emotional communities" seeking shared responses to shared traumas, elites seeking security by pooling the resources of shared wealth and privilege, marginalized men forming gangs, and towns taking up arms to expel narcos and corrupt politicians (Fisher et al. 2018; Macleod and De Marinis 2018; Stahler-Sholk 2007; Sverdlin 2017). The examples demonstrate that even consciously created "collectives" often are not utopian projects. For instance, wealthy people's withdrawal into secure communities reflects and depends on economic inequality, and towns' armed self-governance can become authoritarian. Indeed, violence itself can be part of a collective, if maladaptive, reaction against corrupt governance and entrenched inequality (Pansters 2012). Therapeutic interventions that seek to rehabilitate the family as collective might also involve critique of collectives, including the Mexican nation as a fundamentally colonial enterprise

(Pritzker and Duncan 2019). Further, collectivist responses exist alongside, and often intermingle with, the individualizing, capitalistic destabilization wrought by current crisis and its roots in neoliberal political, economic, and cultural shifts that increase inequality (Valencia Triana 2012).

The people profiled in this book similarly experienced efforts toward collective aid as ambivalent rather than simply empowering. Participation in HIM was not a panacea for the complex sociostructural problems facing Cuernavaca. Further, it sometimes created life difficulties (such as accusations of infidelity) alongside opportunities to enact desired identities and further collective well-being. Yet this case and those discussed earlier reflect the persistence of ideas of personhood as fundamentally collective amid adaptation to neoliberal government reforms and destabilizing violence in Mexico. Using the concept of collective biologies can help us to understand the simultaneously biological and social natures of these collectives and the embodied consequences of their members' engagement in these varied forms of responsibility.

IDENTIFYING COLLECTIVE BIOLOGIES

The collective biologies approach is thus useful for understanding a specific form of embodied relationality. Anthropologists, often writing against the naturalization of individualistic ideologies of personhood in colonizer societies of Europe and North America, have long sought to describe the varied contexts in which people see personhood as fundamentally relational and, further, to identify how relationships inhere into discrete yet nonindividual bodies (see, e.g., Bonnemère 2018; Conklin and Morgan 1996; Viveiros de Castro 1998). This includes mutually transformative relationships among humans and nonhumans (see, e.g., Govindrajan 2018; Haraway 2008; Lupton 2019; Nading 2014; Porter 2019; Roy 2017; Tsing 2015). The concept of collective biology discussed here is intended to identify one specific form of this broader set of diverse experiences of relationality. It refers specifically to the embodied interrelationships created by the shared experience of belonging to a discrete, culturally identified collective.

This means that collective biologies are context-specific. While from an anthropological viewpoint people are always fundamentally interrelated, they do not all believe themselves to be parts of broader biosocial collectives. For example, "the family" may or may not be productively understood as a collective biology. Whether it is depends on the kind of relatedness family members expect to have. As this book shows, this concept fit well with the expectations of enduring, embodied interrelatedness over time that

HIM participants and their partners expected to experience with their own spouses and children. The concept of collective biology also seems appropriate for some people's experiences within Confucian societies, where ideas of one's place in literal and metaphorical families are central to personhood and its embodiment throughout the life course (see, e.g., Zhao 2014).

In such contexts, theorizing family interrelatedness as collective biology could be productive. Regarding the study of care for people with disabilities in China, Zhiying Ma (2019) argues that attending to the family as a key unit of analysis reveals the "non-individualistic, family focused, and gendered configurations of disability, which seem to be the rule rather than the exception for much of the world." I would add that attention to this unit of analysis as a collective biology could reveal how family members' embodied actions influence their relatives' simultaneously biological and social well-being. Further, families, paid caregiver-and-recipient dyads, and others linked by care and interdependence might productively be understood as collective biologies even in contexts in which cultural emphasis on relationality is marginalized or emphasis on individuality is dominant (see, e.g., Buch 2018; Pollak 2018; Selbekk et al. 2018). This analytic can be useful for understanding the embodiment of interrelatedness in any case where people themselves believe that they and a specific other or set of others form a nonindividual unit. "Collective biology" is thus an etic term that can be used to theorize any relationships that people emically understand to entail multiple individuals whose physical and social well-being is interlinked.

In short, the notion of collective biologies can be used to identify and analyze a specific form of interrelationship related to the belief that one is part of a specific collective, rather than to describe the general human experience of relationality. People might disagree about what collectives, if any, exist in their particular context or what the nature or definition of those collectives might be. Collective biologies are not natural or stable categories. Instead, they characterize some people's lived, embodied, and interrelated experiences of acknowledged membership in greater-than-individual social bodies. Which collective biologies exist and who is included in them thus depends on perspective; HIM participants who discussed "Mexicanness" implicitly understood themselves to be part of a national-level collective biology in ways that are not only not shared, but are actively critiqued, by many people in Mexico who identify as Indigenous or Afro-Mexican.

It is critical to acknowledge and trace the evolving social construction of these categories of collectivity for the concept of collective biology to be useful. Beyond identifying cases in which people believe that they make up collectives, this could include proposing the development of new ideologies of interrelatedness. This seems productive in areas of cultural debate and disagreement about the existing and ideal experience of interrelatedness and of embodied personhood. For example, understanding maternal-fetal relationships as collective biologies could provide a way to conceptualize the social and biological experiences of emergent multiplicity during pregnancy without naturalizing culturally specific and politically fraught ideologies of fetal personhood (Howes-Mischel 2016; Morgan 1996).

Overall, as anthropologists continue to innovate new ways to theorize experiences and effects of interconnectedness with beings and structures, within as well as beyond individuals (cf. Solomon 2016), the concept of collective biologies provides a way to identify and analyze discrete yet non-individual units of analysis that people identify as specific sets of relationships that matter for their lives, health, and well-being. Thus, this concept offers an additional analytic for achieving the complex analyses of embodied interrelatedness that are central to the anthropological project.

Using the Collective Biologies Approach beyond Cultural Anthropology

IN BIOCULTURAL RESEARCH

In this analysis I have focused on people's narrative accounts of simultaneously physical and social experiences as fundamental to their research participation. This methodology enabled me to identify the unanticipated finding that became the cornerstone of this book: that HIM participants and their partners understood themselves as elements of nonindividual, biosocial bodies, which they hoped to aid physically as well as socially through medical research participation. Like any set of methods, my approach has provided a view of the world made more productive by acknowledgement of its partiality. Donna Haraway (1988) famously argued that all knowledge is "situated" in a context of creation, and that accounting for that context in analysis strengthens rather than undermines the utility of the findings that emerge. Here I have been able to analyze the social aspects of a biosocial phenomenon, such as people's hopes and expectations that men's HIM involvement would foster positive, embodied changes for others. As part of a broader project of understanding health issues more usefully by attending to the intersection of their social and biological aspects (see, e.g., Haenssgen et al. 2018), I hope that scholars will continue to use ethnographic methods to identify context-specific collective biologies and investigate their health and social consequences.

Such findings could also enable the use of additional methodologies to assess the physical aspects of relationships between individual action and collective biologies. While mixed methodologies, too, provide a partial view of the phenomenon under study, including biological methods in the study of collective biology could link peoples' experiences of their interrelated health and well-being to identification of related physical changes. Several approaches exist that incorporate biological methods with understandings of variables under study as context-specific and contingent and could thus take culturally specific nonindividual bodies as objects of study.

For example, feminist inquiries into the material world from varied disciplines provide models for such investigation. They include practices of biology in which biomedical assessments (see, e.g., Fausto-Sterling 2005) and experimental lab methods (see, e.g., Van Anders 2013) are applied to variables such as sex and gender—and, potentially, nonindividual bodies—which researchers understand as context-contingent, embodied constructs rather than universal natural facts. Biocultural anthropological methods would be similarly useful for understanding the physical aspects of collective biology. These methods vary in type but are unified by the aim of assessing the material aspects of complexly biosocial phenomena while maintaining an understanding of those phenomena as the contingent outcomes of human histories (Goodman and Leatherman 2010; Zuckerman and Martin 2016). Bioethnographic methods, which combine "data derived from biological and ethnographic methods" to meet similar goals while facilitating collaboration from both the bio and social sides of the analytic equation, offer the possibility of combining the ethnographic and bioscientific elements of such a project (Roberts and Sanz 2018: 749). All these approaches lend themselves to the study of biosociality on the level of the nonindividual body.

Using such approaches to study collective biologies could facilitate investigation of the health consequences of membership in marginalized and oppressed social bodies. A wealth of research reveals the biological harm of social assignment to marginalized groups, such as racial groups, on aspects of biology, from epigenetics to reproduction and heart disease (see, e.g., Mullings 2005; Quinlan et al. 2016; Shim 2014; Thayer and Kuzawa 2011; Williams and Collins 1995). Researchers seeking to unify biological and social-science perspectives seek to show that, and assess how, these harms are not simply determined by individual biology (see, e.g., Krieger 2012; Meloni et al. 2018).

As discussed in the introduction, anthropologists argue that racial categories are not scientifically valid; instead, they reflect social groupings believed to be biologically determined but, instead, are linked through shared social experiences that can then influence people's health and life chances (Fuentes et al. 2019). Thus, researchers have worked to show that in cases of health disparities related to racial and other groupings, it is, in fact, the collective social experience of shared hardship and discrimination that then influences group members' bodies in similar, harmful ways. For example, this is apparent in Clarence Gravlee's (2009) foundational findings from Puerto Rico that people's assignment to discriminated-against racial categories, rather than their actual genetic ancestry, correlated with their risk for heart disease. Such cases demonstrate that shared experiences of discrimination, rather than a shared racial biology, drive race-based health disparities and trends.

The concept of collective biologies could be helpful in making such arguments, not just for race, but for other biosocial categories, such as sex and gender, which too often are taken to be discrete biological variables in medical research (cf. Springer et al. 2012). This approach provides a way of describing the kinds of shared biological consequences created by shared social experience and relatedness, without taking the cause of that relatedness as natural, essential, or biologically determined.

IN BIOSCIENTIFIC RESEARCH

Collective, rather than just individual, biologies could be also productive objects of study in biomedical research. Biomedical researchers often take individual bodies as an unquestioned, natural unit of analysis. This assumption means that they can collect only data on biological changes within individual bodies. This is a limitation that impedes scientific discovery in two key ways. First, it limits the questions biomedical research can ask. Second, it reproduces social inequalities within research practice by naturalizing culturally specific conceptions of what counts as a possible unit of analysis. For example, Aidan Seale-Feldman's (2019) study of competing medical and lay interpretations of "mass hysteria" among young rural Nepalese women shows that medical insistence on taking individuals as the unit of analysis not only obscured key aspects of this collective illness experience, but it also perpetuated diagnoses that reflected gender, class, and ethnic inequalities.

The collective biologies approach can rectify this by opening more objects of analysis up to bioscientific study. Instead of focusing only on individual bodies, researchers could identify multiple individual and nonindividual bodies recognized in a specific context that might be affected by a particular health issue. They could then systematically investigate the consequences of the issue under study at multiple levels of scale. Basically, this perspective can transform "the body" and "the human subject" from assumed constants to variables in medical research.

This approach has two key benefits. First, it can enable researchers to ask questions about how both individual and an array of context-specific nonindividual bodies are affected by a person's health behavior. This will generate biological knowledge that is more faithful to participants' lived, complexly biosocial realities. Second, this approach can help biomedical researchers include phenomena in their analyses that currently are often seen only as confounding variables. When biomedical research begins from the assumption that its unit of analysis is only the individual body, the influence of participants' interpersonal experiences on study outcomes (e.g., their compliance with study protocols or report of study outcomes) poses only difficulties for data standardization (Scott et al. 2011). However, if these collaborative phenomena were explicitly made part of an aspect of a study investigating the key collective biologies in which participants were enmeshed, they could be explicitly assessed and incorporated into analysis.

I am suggesting that nuanced biomedical research could ask scientific questions about collective as well as individual bodies, as well as quantitatively assess the biological consequences of individuals' enmeshment in these nonindividual bodies. To do this, researchers would need to take participants' understandings of which collective biologies they make up, and how, seriously as biological data. At the research design phase, investigators could determine the range of nonindividual bodies to which potential participants belong simply by asking whom they hope their participation will directly benefit. The number and nature of these bodies will depend on local culture. However, their cultural determination does not mean they are not also biologically real. Embodied social interactions (from sex to caregiving) between the people who act in accordance with the belief that they form parts of these larger wholes will influence both individual- and group-level biologies.

Knowing that, medical researchers can decide which of these bodies they wish to investigate. They could design studies to generate data about both a certain type of people's individual biologies and their relationships to biological changes in specific, salient collective biologies. Even if medical researchers choose to focus only on individual biologies, they could systematically investigate the biosocial effects of participants' memberships in those broader bodies on their individual biologies. These effects could range from alteration in biomarkers to encouragement of study compliance or noncompliance. Put simply, by taking human subjects' experiences of interrelatedness with others seriously as important biological information, and not just sociocultural ephemera, biomedical researchers can ask more accurate questions about more kinds of bodies.

This approach would enable biomedical study of sets of relationships already identified as salient in the field of public health, such as the role of "men as partners" rather than women or men as individuals in reproductive health care (see, e.g., Wegner et al. 1998; Wentzell and Inhorn 2014). The value in widening the analytic lens in this way is demonstrated by the analysis presented in this book, which used the HIM case to demonstrate the concrete effects of ostensibly individual medical research on nonindividual biologies and the people that constitute them. While this analysis focused on health and social behavior that has physical effects, medical researchers could assess these interactions with a biological lens. Ignoring this interrelatedness in medical research is akin to studying the function of a single organ without ever assessing how it interacts with other parts of anatomy or biochemistry.

The key to assessing nonindividual biologies in biomedical research is treating "body" as a term to define specifically for each research question and site, rather than just a synonym for "individual." Explicitly defining nonindividual units of analysis is already routine practice for scientists who study closely interlinked ecosystems, from coral reefs to forests. Their thinking has spurred an ecological turn that is currently happening within human biology, as well as highlighted by increasing study of the microbiome as central to human health (Lorimer 2019). Such research has required the reconceptualization of human bodies from individual entities to "holobionts," or "ecological unit[s] made up of symbiotic assemblages" (Benezra 2018: n.p.). This shift from individual body to ecosystem as unit of analysis offers a model for understanding embodied interrelationships that include, but are not limited to, humans (Fuentes 2019). Here I have focused this kind of thinking to understand interrelationships of care among multiple humans. If we can understand the human body as a unit bounding a biologically linked assemblage of mammal and microbiota, we can understand a collective biology as a unit bounding an assemblage of particular humans (who, in turn, are assemblages themselves).

Adopting this approach requires advances in both the philosophy and practical tools of bioscience. Simply thinking in terms of ecologies will not change the cultural assumptions and philosophies that animate scientific practice. For example, efforts to understand human biology as context-specific can slide easily into scientifically invalid and socially damaging assertions of essential racial or national difference (Niewöhner and Lock 2018; Stöckelová and Trnka 2020; Yates-Doerr 2017). Similarly, epigenetic thinking about the role of environment on fetal health has not mitigated the sexist and neoliberal assignment of individual responsibility for that health to pregnant women (Ford 2019; Valdez 2018). To avoid such pitfalls, bioscientific study of the health of collective human biologies requires the denaturalization of Western cultural assumptions about personhood—including the emphasis on individuality—that have become the unchallenged philosophical building blocks of biomedical research and practice worldwide. Doing so would further existing efforts to advance bioscience and improve patient care by identifying and challenging the importation of racist and colonialist ideologies of personhood into scientific practice (Radin 2018).

Methodologically, this move requires the development of study designs that reflect this philosophical shift. Such designs could scale up the now accepted scientific understanding of humans as nonindividual assemblages at the molecular level, applying this logic to account for nonindividuality at the biosocial level. For example, clinical research designs could assess changes in collective human biologies conceptualized as holobionts rather than as aggregates of individuals, as they are currently understood in public health (Mason 2018). Social-science and ecological studies of the health consequences of interspecies entanglements offer models for this kind of analysis (Nading 2013), which could be used to think about human collectives in their structural and cultural contexts. Adding the concept of "collective biology" would enable researchers to identify bounded groups of interrelated people to clearly define and assess changes within a nonindividual body under study.

Changing scientific paradigms and practice is difficult. Yet if medical researchers sought to investigate nonindividual human biologies, the next step of identifying whether and which specific collective biologies exist in a particular setting would be relatively simple. At this stage, it is important to underscore that the concept of collective biology is not intended to reference general forms of interrelatedness among humans. Instead, it references discrete biosocial entities that require cultural recognition to exist, since social ideas and practices of relatedness mediate members' physical effects on the whole. The analysis presented here provides a model for how to identify context- and time-specific collective biologies by using qualitative methods to identify the specific biosocial entities that some people understand themselves to constitute.

In the cases presented in this book, participants were quite explicit about the idea that individual health behavior would affect others' embodied well-being. My inspiration to use the term "collective biology" for this phenomenon came from Ricardo, the retired danzón enthusiast, who sought to "participate in programs that benefit health—individual or collective" (see chapter 5). Taking such participants' leads, I then sought to identify the boundaries and dynamics of the collectives participants understood themselves to constitute. I did so by first noting the forms of personhood and relationship that they identified as relevant, such as Mexicanness, machismo/anti-machismo, and marriage, and then using insights from the social-science and history literatures to understand the more implicit conceptions of personhood, relatedness, and identity adhering to these descriptors.

Social-science findings suggest that medical research staff often already have information about individual participants' enmeshment in broader collective biologies (see, e.g., Epstein 1996; Geissler 2011; Geissler et al. 2008). This was exemplified in Michael Montoya's (2011) ethnography of the scientific study of genomic susceptibility to disease among U.S. Latinx communities. While the research designers defined relatedness at the level of DNA similarity among individuals, study participants and front-line staff understood participants to be related in biologically salient ways through kinship, rootedness in place, and shared histories of culture and racialized marginalization. Montoya showed that context-based ideas of belonging and experiences of need influenced study recruitment but were then written out of scientific analysis. As Montoya demonstrates, accounting for this biosocial interrelatedness could have revealed points of similarity and difference between the group of people with a shared genetic ancestry that researchers sought to identify and the group they ended up actually studying: people experiencing shared health consequences of being "Latino/a" in one part of the U.S.-Mexico borderlands. In such scientific research, conceptualizing the group under study as a collective biology could facilitate incorporating knowledge about the biosocial consequences of experiences of interrelatedness into the research design and analysis itself. Making collective biologies the objects of research can thus be a tool for understanding the embodied consequences of group belonging that avoids naturalizing scientifically invalid and socially problematic racial categories.

As Montoya's example shows, front-line biomedical research staff often informally develop the contextual knowledge needed to incorporate participants' experiences of belonging in nonindividual bodies into research design, and thus to ask research questions about collective, as well as individual, biologies. In cases where this knowledge is lacking, it can be obtained through basic use of the social-science method of semistructured interviewing. Put simply, medical researchers can ask people. In writing for doctors about how to account for the ways patients' cultural identities influence their health and health behavior—without resorting to stereotypes—the anthropologist and physician Arthur Kleinman proposes a series of simple questions to identify patients' explanatory model of their illness. Most basically, he proposes that doctors ask what patients think is wrong, hope for, and fear about the condition and its treatment (Kleinman and Benson 2006). Others have elaborated on this suggestion, calling for clinicians to also ask about and learn to identify the ways that structural factors (such as the reliance on exhausting low-wage labor that makes it hard both to afford transportation to the clinic and to find time to cook healthy meals) influence people's health experiences and behavior (Metzl and Hansen 2014). Medical and health research professionals could use a similar approach for identifying the collective biologies their intended research participants might constitute. They could simply ask who participants hope their health behavior might benefit, and how, to identify the interrelationships they experience between their biological states and those of others. These sets of interrelationships, in turn, make up the collective biologies in which they live. These biologies are already involved in and influenced by medical research assessing individual bodies, even if researchers are not yet accounting for them.

IN ETHICS OVERSIGHT OF MEDICAL RESEARCH

The understanding that individuals' research participation can also affect nonindividual, collective biologies can also improve the ethical oversight of biomedical research. This concept provides a way to systematize and operationalize insights from the "empirical turn" in bioethics. This is a move away from relying on universalized ethical norms and toward attending to the ways that diverse real-world contexts, constraints, and relationships differently influence medical decision making, as well as the fundamental ideals of ethics and personhood on which people base such decisions (Hoffmaster 2018).

For instance, one key insight from this approach is the knowledge that Western medical practice is based on culturally specific ideas of ethics and personhood that often conflict with local ideas in the sites to which it is globalized. This individualistic focus may not reflect local ideas about how people should make decisions (e.g., by deciding as a family) and can also obscure the roles that structural inequalities play in participants' experiences (Fisher 2013; Kleinman 1995; Marshall et al. 1994; Muller 1994). Such insights have inspired calls in social science for "situated ethics" that account for nonindividual political, historic, economic, and cultural factors (Molyneux and Geissler 2008). They have also spawned recent efforts in the field of bioethics to better understand collectivist societies by distinguishing autonomy from individualism through a focus on "relational ethics" (Jennings 2016; Rajtar 2018).

This approach can help bioethicists assess how people's common experiences of living for others, demonstrated in HIM participants' experiences and many other social settings, influence their health behavior and the embodied consequences that behavior has for others (see, e.g., Al-Mohammad 2010). It highlights the centrality of relationships to people's practices of "ordinary," daily-life ethics (Das 2012), such as people's efforts to enhance the well-being of others as they simultaneously strive to live out specific, socially appropriate types of relationships and as they relate to the economic, political, and other structures that constrain them (cf. Folayan et al. 2019; Zabiliūtė 2020).

Yet within the practice of bioethics a gap exists between practitioners' increasing agreement that it is necessary to account for the social consequences of research participation, on individual and other levels of scale, and pragmatic guidance about how to do so. Calls to account for the social aspects of research participation often come without methodological instructions (Jordan and Gray 2018). Further, they tend to reductively frame the "social" as a realm that is separate from—rather than intertwined with—the biological changes directly under study. This leads to widespread failure to include easily imaginable and detectable consequences of medical research beyond the individual biological level in consent documents and oversight (cf. Gilbertson et al. 2018).

The findings and recommendations here can serve as one source of such guidance. Reframing "social consequences" as biosocial impacts on collective biologies provides a way forward. If ethics overseers seek to identify the key nonindividual bodies of which research participants form parts, and assess the biosocial consequences of individuals' participation for those bodies, they can more accurately assess the benefits and risks of participation for the bodies actually affected by the pursuit of research in a specific setting. While identifying the "social consequences" of a study might seem an impossibly vast and diffuse task for biomedical researchers and Institutional Review Board staff, assessing the embodied social consequences participation might have for a set of specific, named collective biologies to which a participant belongs is a clearer ask.

The analysis done in this book provides a model for identifying the major collective biologies impacted by a medical research study, as well as the benefits and harms they face from their members' participation in the research. In this case, the main finding was one of unexpected benefit to the couples' and families' bodies, and—participants hoped—to the implicitly and aspirationally mestizo Mexican social body. The HIM participants and their loved ones incorporated research participation into efforts to make health and social gains on levels from the individual to the societal, which were visible from the multiscalar view but would be invisible from an atomistic conception of human subjects' experience. In short, the application of the concept of collective biology to identify the specific, nonindividual bodies affected by men's HIM participation provides a model for identifying other collective biologies affected by other research projects.

IN PUBLIC HEALTH PRACTICE

Understanding how people hope their individual actions will influence their collective biologies, and having the ability to assess these influences quantitatively, can also aid public health practice. Specifically, using this approach can facilitate public health workers' understandings, identification, and promotion of desired health behavior. The findings presented here show that men's individual participation in the HIM study had direct, embodied, and intentional health consequences for their partners, children, and peers. These findings ranged from identifying women's need for cervical cancer screening, ability to focus more resources on children's health care, and promotion of a "culture of prevention" intended to encourage others to get checkups. They demonstrate that health interventions such as testing for sexually transmitted infections (STI) have a range of biological consequences for members of broader collective biologies, not just the person tested and those to whom that person might transmit infection. By accounting for this reality, health workers can better promote interventions such as STI testing and more faithfully assess its health consequences for nonindividual as well as individual bodies. While this book has focused on medical research involving STI testing, these insights could apply to any health behavior.

Beyond generating findings that could assist with the social aspects of health projects, analysis of the role that membership in specific collective biologies plays for health outcomes can inform the provision of medical care and testing via public health programs. Health projects often fall short when they are based on the generalization of knowledge derived from a specific setting. For example, the use of HPV vaccines against the viral genotypes found to be most prevalent and harmful in the global North might not be the best way to prevent cervical cancer in regions where other viral strains are more prevalent (Towghi 2013). Similarly, behavioral health interventions such as self-screening for breast cancer might not work well when promoted outside of the specific "screening ecology" in which they were developed (Burke 2014). Designers of large-scale public health interventions could make better-informed choices based on more nuanced conceptions of generalizability, which would be inherent to medical research attending to collective, rather than only individual, biologies.

IN UNDERSTANDING SURVEILLANCE MEDICINE AND SELF-SURVEILLANCE

The case of HPV testing analyzed here also demonstrates the utility of the collective biologies approach for understanding the biosocial consequences of surveillance medicine more broadly. Longitudinal, observational medical research has effects similar to those of this increasingly widespread form of health care, in which growing numbers of people are defined as "at-risk" and watched for precursors of disease (Armstrong 1995; Twine et al. 2017). This has transformed medical practice, as people are increasingly tested for biomarkers of risk for a wide variety of diseases, then tasked with monitoring that risk and ideally reducing it through healthy behavior. This medical emphasis goes hand in hand with the proliferation of forms of surveillance worldwide, from growing reliance on medical research participation as a source of resources (Fisher 2020; Nguyen 2009; Petryna 2005; Towghi and Vora 2014) to self-surveillance and monitoring of health activities with tools such as Fitbits (Lupton 2016; Lyon et al. 2012; Race 2012; R. Sanders 2017). Understanding oneself as a source of health data that should be collected and assessed has become a way to seek health while also meeting cultural norms of personal responsibility.

Such practices seem focused on individual bodies and often rely on technologies designed within societies that emphasize individualism. Yet investigating the impacts of self-surveillance on collective biologies can reveal how monitoring individual bodily change can be a deliberate effort to positively affect the bodies and lives of the others with whom one is enmeshed. As shown in this book, engaging in health surveillance via medical research participation can be a way to seek positive changes in diverse life arenas, such as spiritual practice, work, and parenting. Assessing the impacts of individual surveillance on collective biologies can reveal its nonindividual consequences, ranging far beyond the clinical realm.

Conclusion

This book analyzes an understudied form of health research that sheds light on the broader global phenomenon of increasing medical and self-surveillance. It provides a model for understanding how people adopt these trends in the context of globalization of neoliberal governance and practices to seek to live out self-consciously modern gender, racial, family, and health behavior amid destabilizing crises and the clash of individualizing global and collectivist local ideas about who people are and should be. I hope that the HIM participants' and their partners' efforts to help the broader collective biologies in which they are enmeshed through men's research participation offer a model that researchers can use to analyze the complex interactions of all these forces in other contexts. I further hope that my analysis here inspires and provides an approach for designing quantitative biomedical, as well as qualitative, investigations of the effects of specific human experiences within these broader trends on collective as well as individual biologies.

Many of the world's people understand their membership in collectives to be fundamental to their health and their selfhood, and they make health decisions based on the desire to aid collectives rather than just their personal biologies. My goal in this book has been to theorize that phenomenon in the case of the Mexican HIM study, with three aims in mind. The first was to understand how specifically Mexican ideologies of race and gender, in a context of change, crisis, and valorization of modernity, influenced people's experiences of globalized medical research. The second was to provide an analytic model for understanding the nonindividual aspects of medical research participation. Third, I have sought to build on that ethnographic analysis to make a case for the utility of this perspective for biomedical, as well as sociocultural, research. It is an obvious truth that many of the worlds' people understand themselves primarily within the web of relationships they inhabit, rather than envisioning selfhood as fundamentally individual. Yet assessing the relationships between individual actions and changes in broader, biosocial bodies can seem daunting. The concept of collective biologies, and its application in this book, provides one approach for understanding these interactions and our complexly biosocial realities.

Methods

I learned about the Human Papillomavirus Infection in Men (HIM) study by chance as I did fieldwork for an earlier book, based in the Urology Department of the Cuernavaca Instituto Mexicano del Seguro Social (IMSS) hospital in 2007–2008, on men's experiences of decreased erectile function. I had found that field site with the help of the director of the research unit that administered the HIM study, who kindly offered me the use of a computer in the unit's offices to type up my field notes.

Every afternoon I joined the staff for lunch, then typed up my morning's interview notes. It was there that I heard about the new men's human papillomavirus (HPV) study they had begun and about their recruitment plans and experiences with their first participants. As an anthropologist I was amazed by the amount of data being collected from HIM participants, the potential social import of experiences such as being diagnosed with an asymptomatic but potentially stigmatizing sexually transmitted infection (STI), and the fact that no one was asking what I considered the most interesting questions about how those experiences affected men's lives. The study staff graciously agreed to let me ask those questions. They offered logistical support for my research and agreed that they would not need to know my findings until publication so as not to influence my analysis. The Cuernavaca HIM staff asked nothing of me but mutually beneficial joint work on other HPV-related research projects where my qualitative analysis skills would be helpful but were not part of the HIM study itself (León-Maldonado et al. 2016; Wentzell et al. 2016).

I sought to study the consequences of men's medical research enrollment over time for participants and the broader biosocial bodies to which they belonged. My goal was to understand how people collaborated to incorporate this seemingly individual, biologically focused experience into their broader relationships and ongoing efforts to be particular kinds of people amid dramatic social change. So I took couples rather than individual male participants as my main unit of analysis. Couples interviews were important for understanding the consequences of longitudinal study participation in a society that emphasizes family belonging as central to identity (Lomnitz-Adler 2001). I focused on heterosexual partnerships for both practical and theory-driven reasons: There were very few men who identified as having male partners in the HIM questionnaires, and I was interested in how changing ideologies of heterosexual marriage and masculinity influenced couples' study experiences.

This method of interviewing couples also promised to generate rich data on the relationship between medical experience and spouses' individual and jointly constructed identities, as I found in my own, prior Cuernavaca-based research on men's changing sexual function (Wentzell 2013). While that research focused on men experiencing decreased erectile function, research participants sometimes asked for their wives to join in our conversations. The resulting interactions showed me that talking with couples together could reveal how people collaborate to make sense of health experiences and to live out shared couples' identities through them, as well as how they debate and assert who "we" are and want to be. This focus on couples also made sense since STI testing and positive diagnoses in men directly affected their sexual partners, in terms of both health risks, such as cervical cancer, and social risks, such as blame, guilt, and the specter of infidelity.

Throughout this book, I draw on data from these interviews with couples to make claims that Mexican HIM participants and their partners experienced men's medical research participation as relevant for the embodied well-being of greater-than-individual entities. It is important to note that while the methodology of interviewing couples encouraged participants to highlight experiences of collectivity in their narratives, this finding is not simply an artifact of the methods used. I know this for two reasons. First, I interviewed comparison groups of men and women individually, and they voiced similar themes. Second, unpublished exploratory interviews I did with male participants in the Tampa, Florida, arm of the HIM study revealed dramatically different experiences. In both Cuernavaca and Tampa, staff invited those HIM participants who seemed most enthusiastic about the study to talk with me. Yet unlike the Cuernavacan men, the Americans characterized participation as a fundamentally individual experience and often did not even mention their HIM experiences to their partners. I am thus confident that the methods used here served to gather data on context-specific, relational aspects of HIM participation in Mexico.

This approach also meets calls from anthropology and public health to focus on couples, rather than individuals, in studies of fundamentally interpersonal sexual health issues (Hirsch et al. 2009; Schensul et al. 2006). It also requires specific methodological and ethical considerations. Most basically, interviewers must use techniques to encourage talk from all participants—for example, making discursive space for one partner's response to another's "scene stealing" (Arksey 1996). Since such interviews provide particularly nuanced information about the gendered ways in which couples negotiate sexual health issues, they can also raise difficult emotions that interviewers must be particularly conscious of to foster dialogue without creating stress or fueling interpersonal difficulty (Gerrits 2018). The interviewer's attention to such dynamics enhances not just participants' comfort but also the quality of subsequent data analysis. The emotional flows and interactions of narrative construction in interviews are themselves key data (Hoffmann 2007). Attention to this, as well as reflexivity about the role the researcher's identity and behavior play in shaping the context-specific joint narrative resulting from the interview, is necessary for analysis (Gerrits 2018; Seale et al. 2008).

I knew that studying couples' experiences of men's HIM participation would provide a way to understand people's responses to changing ideals for masculinity and marriage, in a cultural context where both sexual and health practice have long been contested life arenas in which people associate actions with good and bad personhood. What I did not anticipate when I began this study was that a crisis of violence would arise that would fundamentally alter the research participants' lives. As the crisis unfolded over time, this project came to investigate how people incorporated their sexual and health practices into efforts to care for and protect their loved ones at a time of insecurity and to seek to help move their society forward as they worried that it was disintegrating around them. This unexpected development demonstrates the utility of studying longitudinal research as a way to understand the consequences of medical research participation. Its long time span enables study of the interrelationships that develop between medical research experiences and other life experiences that unfold over time, especially in terms of participants' processual relationships with their ever-changing bodies, loved ones, and structural circumstances. This longitudinal focus was especially helpful for understanding the gendered and ethical consequences of STI research and surveillance, given the long time span between HPV infection and symptoms and the long time course over which participants received and disclosed positive results and their spouses reacted to these events.

Participants in my anthropological study were recruited by HIM staff from a pool of male participants who invited their female romantic partners to participate in a planned, though never executed, medical study of HPV in women. Since the group of spouses who volunteered included men who felt comfortable participating in STI surveillance and qualitative interviews regarding that surveillance together with their wives, they cannot be viewed as representative of the Cuernavaca or even HIM study populations. Instead, this book examines the experiences of a particular group of people who wanted to participate in medical research as a family affair. Even male HIM study participants who had not expressed interest in their partners' involvement in the women's study, and thus were not included in the present study, might have had different experiences of medical research participation. For instance, they might have kept test results or study events secret from partners, experiencing HIM participation as more individual—or simply less meaningful—than the men discussed here.

So this study population reveals the experiences of medical research participants who chose to incorporate that experience into their daily lives and relationships. It includes thirty-one male-female couples, as well as comparison groups of twelve women alone and ten men alone, who participated in a series of three annual semi-structured Spanish-language interviews, undertaken between 2010 and 2013, with follow-up with some participants in 2015. I also did annual interviews with HIM physicians and the clinical manager of the HIM study to learn about study procedures and events and to get their views on participants' experiences. Annual interviews worked well as a methodology for studying a longitudinal research project, since they provided a view of change over time and a comparison between earlier and later experiences, as well as a view over time of couples' experiences in relationship to changing context. While I used the comparison groups to assess whether people spoke differently about their experiences in the presence or absence of their spouses, I found that very similar themes emerged across groups. The only key difference was that people interviewed alone were more likely to discuss considering or committing infidelity; that issue also often arose in couple's interviews but more commonly in the form of accusations or discussions of events that were already known to both partners.

Whenever possible, the HIM staff scheduled my interviews with participants directly after their clinical visits to spare them extra travel. I conducted the interviews in private areas at the HIM research clinics—usually empty examination rooms in the early site and at a shaded table in a walled court-yard at the study's final home. For participants' convenience, I also held some interviews with men at private areas in their workplaces.

I did all interviews in Spanish. They lasted an average of forty-five min-utes. Most participants gave permission for digital recording of interviews for later transcription, and I took written notes to record interview content and nonverbal forms of communication, such as physical contact between spouses. All of the participants signed informed consent forms and were told that their decisions regarding participation in the anthropological study would not impact their HIM study eligibility or treatment. My research protocol was approved by the University of Iowa and IMSS Institutional Review Boards, and all names used here are pseudonyms. As a testament to their familiarity with research documents and interest in the research process, participants tended to read the consent forms closely and have many questions.

The initial interviews collected participants' life, health, and romantic histories and elicited discussion of their HIM study experiences to date, including reasons for enrollment. Subsequent interviews gathered data on participants' changing experiences and ideas over time, addressing their un-derstandings of the HIM study and marital, health, and other key life experi-ences that had occurred since the prior interview. We also discussed recent STI testing results and couples' responses—medical and emotional—to them each year. I designed these interviews in light of best practices in qualitative research on intimate topics, including ordering questions from least to most intimate, demonstrating confidentiality, establishing rapport, and avoiding assumptions (e.g., I used gender-neutral language to avoid suggesting that I expected all participants' sexual partners to be of the opposite sex) (Herdt and Lindenbaum 1992; Parker et al. 2000).

I began each interview with a set of questions to address; after the first year, the questions were personalized to follow up on what we had previ-ously discussed. However, since my goal was to understand how people re-lated study experiences to other daily-life events, and since I was focusing on the relationships that influenced those experiences, the interviews were very open-ended. They went down the conversational paths that participants chose so that I could learn what nonobvious links people drew between study events and daily life. It was through this approach that the unexpected connections participants drew between medical research participation and their experiences of the insecurity crisis were revealed.

Interviews were my main method because they offered these insights and because of the nature of doing research *on* medical research. Interviews were easy to fit into the daily life of the HIM study (which already involved computer-based questionnaires) and made sense as a methodology to the public health researchers who determined my access. Because I was working with medical research participants, maintaining confidentiality was crucial: they had already been guaranteed confidentiality as HIM participants, so I had to be sure not to attempt to engage with participants in public settings in ways that would compromise that. In couples interviews I was also attentive to the ways that people agreed on or debated who "we" were or why "we" enrolled in the study, what study-related experiences meant for them as a family, and who they should try to be as men and women.

However, given my research interest in how people related the study to their broader life experiences, this methodology presented some limitations. Anthropologists famously use participant observation because of the wide gaps between what people think and say they do and their behavior in practice, as well as the fact that narrative data both reflect the specific interpersonal interaction that generates them and capture only a portion of human experience. Thus, I also included observation and participant observation in my methods. I observed daily life in the HIM study by becoming part of it during my time there—working at a computer and taking meal breaks with the other staff members and observing some HIM data collection procedures in which staff and participants engaged. While I do not use those data directly in the present analysis, the experience of being present in a Mexican medical context during the time of the study informed my thinking about life in Cuernavaca at the time of the research project.

I also engaged in participant observation in the daily-life activities of a subset of participants. To honor the need to maintain confidentiality, I used this method only with participants who actively invited me to join them in specific events. As we got to know one another over time, six couples and individuals invited me to visit their homes, eat out, or engage in activities such as exercise classes or multilevel marketing sales work. Evangelical Christian participants were the most likely to extend invitations to me, often inviting me to attend worship services and church-related social events. These participants gave additional verbal consent for me to incorporate my experiences of their lives outside the clinic into my analysis of the social consequences of their HIM involvement. While limited, these experiences provided a window into the ways that people were living out the themes they raised in our interviews in other daily-life arenas.

Data Analysis

In my analysis I sought to understand how participants both jointly and individually incorporated medical study experiences into new or ongoing performances of ethics and identity, and their hopes for change in the collective biologies in which they believed themselves enmeshed. I identified emergent themes, patterns, and changes over time in participants' discussions of study and other life experiences related to these issues in interview and observation notes and transcriptions. Understanding interviews as collaborative encounters that produce narrative as a "cooperative achievement," I employ a constructivist perspective in my analysis of interview data (Linde 1993: 12). This means that I see such data as reflecting people's narrative construction of self in a specific context, rather than a journalistic account of participants' experiences (Jackson 1998; Morris 1995). In this light, couples interviews are especially important for revealing how spouses negotiate and assert both joint and individual identities in a specific setting. Interviews served as a space for participants both to describe their experience and to enact and define who they were trying to be as men, women, parents, spouses, and citizens.

Participants' positionalities and my identity as a white, female, American researcher influenced these interactions. Being a foreign woman might have made men feel more able to express sexual vulnerability to me than they would to a fellow Mexican or man (González-López 2005; Wentzell 2013), although my femaleness might have deterred performances of more traditional aspects of masculinity (Hirsch et al. 2007). It also likely facilitated discussion with female participants (Reinharz and Chase 2002). My foreignness also likely encouraged participants to speak of themselves "as Mexicans" and to explain what being Mexican meant to educate me in the background needed to understand their experiences.

My being a white American also mattered in a particular way. In our conversations, participants both associated the United States with aspirational modernity and wealth and critiqued it as a source of oppressive inequality and promoter of regressively xenophobic politics on the regional stage. In our interviews, participants and their partners expressed these views in explicit comparisons between the United States and Mexico, as well as in their implicit narrative choices, as a response to my nationality. My whiteness led participants to relate to me as a representative of dominant U.S. culture, including their critiques of that culture. While racial difference shaped our interactions, my whiteness and participants' middle-class takes on Mexicanness also involved a kind of similarity, given the implicit goal of mestizaje aimed toward modernity and population whitening inherent to Mexican discussions of "good citizenship." My status as a researcher clearly created such kinship, with participants in medical and academic careers understanding me to be from a similar work milieu.

However, both my identity and the context of couples interviews likely led participants to avoid certain topics, as when men admitted to infidelity privately to me or in HIM questionnaires but denied it to their wives. Participants' perception of me as affiliated with the HIM study (despite my reminders that I was an independent researcher) also influenced our conversations. While these limitations mean that some of ways in which medical research experiences shaped participants' lives remain unknown, the interview data overall reveal the context-specific, collaborative ways that people related men's HIM participation to their roles in broader biosocial bodies.

It was also the case that the HIM study itself made certain kinds of experiences speakable. In Mexico, the ethnographer Héctor Carillo (2002) has documented the widespread practice of "sexual silence": strategic vagueness around matters of sexuality that enables evasion of stigma and maintenance of familial respect in the face of nonideal sexual practice. It makes peoples' lives easier but can hamper collection of data on nonideal intimate practices. However, medical frankness is generally valued in urban central Mexico, where, the medical anthropologist Kaja Finkler (1991: xv) argues, "Sickness is not usually regarded as a private matter in Mexican popular culture," and researchers' questioning is usually regarded as a sign of polite interest. Participants in my prior Cuernavaca-based research on men's experiences of decreasing erectile function often stated that they felt able to discuss this potentially stigmatizing issue because we spoke in a clinical context (Wentzell 2013). Based on similar comments from participants in the present study (including those who invited me to participate in daily life activities), it appears that this research site offered some degree of exemption from the sexual silence through which participants might deal with intimate or stigmatizing issues in daily life. This research site thus enables the study of medical research participation as a social phenomenon, as well as the ways that people incorporated sexuality-related practices into unfolding performances of self- and couplehood and efforts to heal broader biosocial bodies as they responded to societal change.

REFERENCES

Abadie, Roberto. 2010. *The Professional Guinea Pig: Big Pharma and the Risky World of Human Subjects*. Durham, NC: Duke University Press.

Adams, Vincanne, and Stacy Leigh Pigg, eds. 2005. *Sex in Development*. Durham, NC: Duke University Press.

Adkins, Lisa. 2001. "Risk Culture, Self-Reflexivity and the Making of Sexual Hierarchies." *Body and Society* 7(1): 35–55.

Adler, Marina. 2012. "Collective Identity Formation and Collective Action Framing in a Mexican 'Movement of Movements.'" *Interface* 4(1): 287–315.

Aguayo Quezada, Sergio, Rodrigo Peña González, and Jorge Ariel Ramírez Pérez. 2014. *Atlas de la seguridad y violencia en Morelos*. Universidad Autónoma del Estado de Morelos and Colectivo de Análisis de la Seguridad con Democracia. https://www.casede.org/PublicacionesCasede/AtlasMorelos.pdf.

Ahearn, Laura M. 2001. *Invitations to Love: Literacy, Love Letters, and Social Change in Nepal*. Ann Arbor: University of Michigan Press.

Alenichev, Arsenii, and Vinh-Kim Nguyen. 2019. "Precarity, Clinical Labour and Graduation from Ebola Clinical Research in West Africa." *Global Bioethics* 30(1): 1–18.

Al-Mohammad, Hayder. 2010. "Towards an Ethics of Being-With: Intertwinements of Life in Post-Invasion Basra." *Ethnos* 75(4): 425–46.

Al-Mohammad, Hayder. 2012. "A Kidnapping in Basra: The Struggles and Precariousness of Life in Postinvasion Iraq." *Cultural Anthropology* 27(4): 597–614.

Alonso, Ana María. 1995. *Thread of Blood: Colonialism, Revolution, and Gender on Mexico's Northern Frontier*. Tucson: University of Arizona Press.

Alonso, Ana María. 2004. "Conforming Disconformity: 'Mestizaje,' Hybridity, and the Aesthetics of Mexican Nationalism." *Cultural Anthropology* 19(4): 459–90.

Amuchástegui Herrera, Ana. 1996. El significado de la virginidad y la iniciación sexual: Un relato de investigación. In *Para comprender la subjetividad: Investigación cualitativa en salud reproductiva y sexualidad*, edited by Ivonne Szasz and Susana Lerner, 137–72. Mexico City: El Colegio de México.

Amuchástegui Herrera, Ana. 1998. "Virginity in Mexico: The Role of Competing Discourses of Sexuality in Personal Experience." *Reproductive Health Matters* 6(12): 105–15.

Amuchástegui Herrera, Ana. 2008. "La masculinidad como culpa esencial: Subjetivación, género y tecnología de sí en un programa de reeducación para hombres violentos." In *II Congreso Nacional los Estudios de Género de los Hombres en México: Caminos andados y nuevos retos en investigación y Acción*. Mexico City.

Amuchástegui Herrera, Ana, and Ivonne Szasz, eds. 2007. *Sucede que me canso de ser hombre*. Mexico City: El Colegio de Mexico.

Arksey, Hilary. 1996. "Collecting Data through Joint Interviews." *Social Research Update* 15(Winter): 1–4.

Armstrong, David. 1995. "The Rise of Surveillance Medicine." *Sociology of Health and Illness* 17(3): 393–404.

Armstrong, Natalie. 2005. "Resistance through Risk: Women and Cervical Cancer Screening." *Health, Risk and Society* 7(2): 161–76.

Armstrong, Natalie. 2019. "Navigating the Uncertainties of Screening: The Contribution of Social Theory." *Social Theory and Health* 17(2): 158–71.

Ávila González, Yanina. 2017. "Transformando la educación: Mujer = madre. In *¡A toda madre! Una mirada multidisciplinaria a las maternidades en México*, edited by Abril Saldaña-Tejeda, Lilia Venegas Aguilera, and Tine Davids, 249–74. Mexico City: Científica.

Benezra, Amber. 2018. "Making Microbiomes." In *Routledge Handbook of Genomics, Health and Society*, edited by Sahra Gibbon, Barbara Prainsack, Stephen Hilgartner, and Janelle Lamoreaux, 283–90. London: Routledge.

Berger, Peter L., and Robert W. Hefner. 2013. *Global Pentecostalism in the 21st Century*. Bloomington: Indiana University Press.

Bertone, Chiara. 2017. "Good and Healthy Parents: Non-Heterosexual Parenting and Tricky Alliances." *Italian Sociological Review* 7(3): 351–67.

Biehl, João, Denise Coutinho, and AnaLuzia Outeiro. 2001. "Technology and Affect: HIV/AIDS Testing in Brazil." *Culture, Medicine and Psychiatry* 25(1): 87–129.

Biruk, Crystal. 2011. "Seeing like a Research Project: Producing 'High-Quality Data' in AIDS Research in Malawi." *Medical Anthropology* 31(4): 347–66.

Biruk, Crystal. 2018. *Cooking Data: Culture and Politics in an African Research World*. Durham, NC: Duke University Press.

Black, Steven P. 2019. "Ethics, Expertise, and Inequities in Global Health Discourses." In *Language and Social Justice in Practice*, edited by Netta Avineri, Laura R. Graham, Eric J. Johnson, Robin Conley Riner, and Jonathan Rosa, 119–27. New York: Routledge.

Bliss, Katherine. 1999. "Paternity Tests: Fatherhood on Trial in Mexico's Revolution of the Family." *Journal of Family History* 24(3): 330–50.

Bonnemère, Pascale. 2018. *Acting for Others: Relational Transformations in Papua New Guinea*. Chicago: HAU.

Braff, Lara. 2013. "Somos Muchos (We Are So Many)." *Medical Anthropology Quarterly* 27(1): 121–38.

Brandes, Stanley. 2002. *Staying Sober in Mexico City*. Austin: University of Texas Press.

Briggs, Laura. 2002. *Reproducing Empire: Race, Sex, Science, and U.S. Imperialism in Puerto Rico*. Berkeley: University of California Press.

Brito, Jaime Luis. 2016. "Y en Cuernavaca se manifiestan contra 'violencia machista.'" *Proceso.com*, April 24. http://www.proceso.com.mx/438374/vivasnosqueremos -contra-acoso-sexual-en-cuernavaca.

Broholm-Jørgensen, Marie, Nina Kamstrup-Larsen, Ann Dorrit Guassora, and Susanne Reventlow et al. 2019. "'It Can't Do Any Harm': A Qualitative Exploration of Accounts of Participation in Preventive Health Checks." *Health, Risk and Society* 21(1–2): 57–73.

Brotherton, P. Sean, and Vinh-Kim Nguyen. 2013. "Revisiting Local Biology in the Era of Global Health." *Medical Anthropology* 32(4): 287–90.

Browner, Carole. 1989. "La producción de la reproducción y la salud de la mujer: Estudio de un caso de Oaxaca, México." *Anales de Antropología* 26: 319–29.

Brusco, Elizabeth. 1993. "The Reformation of Masculinity: Asceticism and Masculinity among Colombian Evangelicals." In *Rethinking Protestantism in Latin America*, edited by Virginia Garrard-Burnett and David Stoll, 143–58. Philadelphia: Temple University Press.

Bruun, Birgitte. 2016. "Foregrounding Possibilities and Backgrounding Exploitation in Transnational Medical Research Projects in Lusaka, Zambia." *Focaal* 74: 54–66.

Buch, Elana D. 2018. *Inequalities of Aging: Paradoxes of Independence in American Home Care*. New York: New York University Press.

Burke, Nancy J. 2014. "Local Biologies and Ecologies of Screening: Tracing the Aftereffects of the 'Shanghai Study.'" *Anthropological Quarterly* 87(2): 497–524.

Butler, Judith. 1990. *Gender Trouble: Feminism and the Subversion of Identity*. New York: Routledge.

Cahn, Peter S. 2008. "Consuming Class: Multilevel Marketers in Neoliberal Mexico." *Cultural Anthropology* 23(3): 429–52.

Cant, Alanna. 2018. "'Making' Labour in Mexican Artisanal Workshops." *Journal of the Royal Anthropological Institute* 24(S1): 61–74.

Careaga Valdez, Gabriel. 1987. *Mitos y realidades de la clase media en México*. Mexico City: Oceano.

Carillo, Héctor. 2002. *The Night Is Young: Sexuality in Mexico in the Time of AIDS*. Chicago: University of Chicago Press.

Carillo, Héctor. 2007. "Imagining Modernity: Sexuality, Policy, and Social Change in Mexico." *Sexuality Research and Social Policy* 4(3): 74–91.

Carlos, Manuel L. 1973. "Fictive Kinship and Modernization in Mexico: A Comparative Analysis." *Anthropological Quarterly* 46(2): 75–91.

Carruth, Lauren. 2018. "The Data Hustle: How Beneficiaries Benefit from Continual Data Collection and Humanitarian Aid Research in the Somali Region of Ethiopia." *Medical Anthropology Quarterly* 32(3): 340–64.

Casper, Monica J., and Laura M. Carpenter. 2009. "Sex, Drugs, and Politics: The HPV Vaccine for Cervical Cancer." In *Pharmaceuticals and Society: Critical Discourses and Debates*, edited by Simon J. Williams, Jonathan Gabe, and Peter Davis, 71–84. Malden, MA: Wiley-Blackwell.

Castor, N. Fadeke. 2017. *Spiritual Citizenship: Transnational Pathways from Black Power to Ifá in Trinidad*. Durham, NC: Duke University Press.

Castro, Roberto. 2001. "'When a Man Is with a Woman, It Feels like Electricity': Subjectivity, Sexuality and Contraception among Men in Central Mexico." *Culture, Health and Sexuality* 3(2): 149–65.

Centers for Disease Control and Prevention. 2013. STD Curriculum for Clinical Educators: Genital Human Papillomavirus (HPV) Module.

Charles, Nicole. 2013. "Mobilizing the Self-Governance of Pre-damaged Bodies: Neoliberal Biological Citizenship and HPV Vaccination Promotion in Canada." *Citizenship Studies* 17(6–7): 770–84.

Charles, Nicole. 2018. "HPV Vaccination and Affective Suspicions in Barbados." *Feminist Formations* 30(1): 46–70.

Chaves, Margarita, and Marta Zambrano. 2006. "From Blanqueamiento to Reindigenización: Paradoxes of Mestizaje and Multiculturalism in Contemporary Colombia." *Revista Europea de Estudios Latinoamericanos y del Caribe/European Review of Latin American and Caribbean Studies* 80: 5–23.

Chavez, Leo R., Juliet M. McMullin, Shiraz I. Mishra, and F. Allan Hubbell. 2001. "Beliefs Matter: Cultural Beliefs and the Use of Cervical Cancer-Screening Tests." *American Anthropologist* 103(4): 1114–29.

Cházaro, Laura. 2005. "Mexican Women's Pelves and Obstetrical Procedures: Interventions with Forceps in Late 19th Century Medicine." *Feminist Review* 79: 100–15.

Cho, Jieun. 2020. "Family in the Ruins of Nuclear Risk." *Anthropology News*, April 29.

Clifford, G. M., S. Gallus, R. Herrero, and N. Muñoz et al. 2005. "Worldwide Distribution of Human Papillomavirus Types in Cytologically Normal Women in the International Agency for Research on Cancer HPV Prevalence Surveys: A Pooled Analysis." *The Lancet* 366(9490): 991–98.

Compaoré, Adélaïde, Susan Dierickx, Fatou Jaiteh, and Alain Nahum et al. 2018. "Fear and Rumours Regarding Placental Biopsies in a Malaria-in-Pregnancy Trial in Benin." *Malaria Journal* 17(1): 425.

Conklin, Beth A., and Lynn M. Morgan. 1996. "Babies, Bodies, and the Production of Personhood in North America and a Native Amazonian Society." *Ethos* 24(4): 657–94.

Consejo Estatal de Población de Morelos. 2013. *Zona metropolitana de Cuernavaca 2013*. Consejo Estatal de Población de Morelos, Cuernavaca. http://www.coespomor .gob.mx/Publicaciones_COESPO/Cuadernillo_zona_metropolitana_Cuernavaca.pdf.

Consejo Nacional de Evaluación de la Política de Desarrollo Social (CONEVAL). 2012. "Informe de pobreza y evaluación en el estado de Morelos 2012." https://www .coneval.org.mx/coordinacion/entidades/Documents/Informes%20de%20po-breza%20y%20evaluaci%C3%B3n%202010-2012_Documentos/Informe%20de%20 pobreza%20y%20evaluaci%C3%B3n%202012_Morelos.pdf.

Cooper, Melinda, and Catherine Waldby. 2014. *Clinical Labor: Tissue Donors and Research Subjects in the Global Bioeconomy*. Durham, NC: Duke University Press.

Crowley-Matoka, Megan. 2016. *Domesticating Organ Transplant: Familial Sacrifice and National Aspiration in Mexico*. Durham, NC: Duke University Press.

Crowley-Matoka, Megan, and Margaret Lock. 2006. "Organ Transplantation in a Globalised World." *Mortality* 11(2): 166–81.

Csordas, Thomas J. 2008. "Intersubjectivity and Intercorporeality." *Subjectivity* 22(1): 110–21.

Daley, Ellen M., Cheryl A. Vamos, Gregory D. Zimet, and Zeev Rosberger et al. 2016. "The Feminization of HPV: Reversing Gender Biases in U.S. Human Papillomavirus Vaccine Policy." *American Journal of Public Health* 106(6): 983–4.

Das, Veena. 2012. "Ordinary Ethics." In *A Companion to Moral Anthropology*, edited by Didier Fassin, 133–49. Malden, MA: John Wiley and Sons.

Davis, Diane E. 2018. "The Routinization of Violence in Latin America: Ethnographic Revelations." *Latin American Research Review* 53(1): 211–16.

Dawley, William. 2018. "From Wrestling with Monsters to Wrestling with God: Masculinities, 'Spirituality,' and the Group-ization of Religious Life in Northern Costa Rica." *Anthropological Quarterly* 91(1): 79–131.

Dawley, William, and Brendan Jamal Thornton. 2018. "New Directions in the Anthropology of Religion and Gender: Faith and Emergent Masculinities." *Anthropological Quarterly* 91(1): 5–23.

de Keijzer, Benno. 2016. "'Sé que debo parar, pero no sé cómo': Abordajes teóricos en torno a los hombres, la salud y el cambio." *Sexualidad, Salud y Sociedad* (22): 278–300.

de la Cadena, Marisol, ed. 2008. *Formaciones de indianidad: Articulaciones raciales, mestizaje y nación en América Latina*. Bogotá: Envión.

Dermott, Esther. 2012. "Poverty versus Parenting: An Emergent Dichotomy." *Studies in the Maternal* 4(2): 1–13.

de Wit, J. B. F., and P. C. G. Adam. 2008. "To Test or Not to Test: Psychosocial Barriers to HIV Testing in High-Income Countries." *HIV Medicine* 9: 20–22.

Dixon, Justin, and Michèle Tameris. 2018. "Clean Blood, Religion, and Moral Triage in Tuberculosis Vaccine Trials." *Medical Anthropology* 37(8): 708–21.

Domínguez-Ruvalcaba, Héctor. 2007. *Modernity and the Nation in Mexican Representations of Masculinity: From Sensuality to Bloodshed*. New York: Palgrave Macmillan.

Douglas, Bronwen. 2003. "Christianity, Tradition, and Everyday Modernity: Towards an Anatomy of Women's Groupings in Melanesia." *Oceania* 74(1–2): 6–23.

Dow, James. 2005. "The Expansion of Protestantism in Mexico: An Anthropological View." *Anthropological Quarterly* 78(4): 827–50.

Dresser, Rebecca. 2002. "The Ubiquity and Utility of the Therapeutic Misconception." *Social Philosophy and Policy* 19(2): 271–94.

Duncan, Whitney L. 2017. "Dinámicas Ocultas: Culture and Psy-sociality in Mexican Family Constellations Therapy." *Ethos* 45(4): 489–513.

Durkheim, Émile. (1912) 2008. *The Elementary Forms of Religious Life*, translated by Joseph Ward Swain. Mineola, NY: Dover.

Elliott, Carl, and Roberto Abadie. 2008. "Exploiting a Research Underclass in Phase 1 Clinical Trials." *New England Journal of Medicine* 358(22): 2316–17.

Epstein, Steven. 1996. *Impure Science: AIDS, Activism, and the Politics of Knowledge*. Berkeley: University of California Press.

Epstein, Steven. 2008a. *Inclusion: The Politics of Difference in Medical Research*. Chicago: University of Chicago Press.

Epstein, Steven. 2008b. "The Rise of 'Recruitmentology': Clinical Research, Racial Knowledge, and the Politics of Inclusion and Difference. *Social Studies of Science* 38(5): 801–32.

Esteinou, Rosario. 2005. "Parenting in Mexican Society." *Marriage and Family Review* 36(3–4): 7–29.

Everett, Margaret, and Michelle Ramirez. 2015. "Healing the Curse of the Grosero Husband: Women's Health Seeking and Pentecostal Conversion in Oaxaca, Mexico." *Journal of Contemporary Religion* 30(3): 415–33.

Fairhead, James, Melissa Leach, and Mary Small. 2006. "Where Techno-science Meets Poverty: Medical Research and the Economy of Blood in the Gambia, West Africa." *Social Science and Medicine* 63(4): 1109–20.

Farmer, Paul. 2002. "Can Transnational Research Be Ethical in the Developing World?" *The Lancet* 360(9342): 1266.

Fausto-Sterling, Anne. 2005. "The Bare Bones of Sex: Part 1—Sex and Gender." *Signs* 30(2): 1491–527.

Fesenmyer, Leslie. 2018. "Pentecostal Pastorhood as Calling and Career: Migration, Religion, and Masculinity between Kenya and the United Kingdom." *Journal of the Royal Anthropological Institute* 24(4): 749–66.

Finkler, Kaja. 1991. *Physicians at Work, Patients in Pain: Biomedical Practice and Patient Response in Mexico*. Boulder, CO: Westview.

Finkler, Kaja. 1994. *Women in Pain: Gender and Morbidity in Mexico*. Philadelphia: University of Pennsylvania Press.

Fisher, Jill A. 2008. *Medical Research for Hire: The Political Economy of Pharmaceutical Clinical Trials*. New Brunswick, NJ: Rutgers University Press.

Fisher, Jill A. 2013. "Expanding the Frame of 'Voluntariness' in Informed Consent: Structural Coercion and the Power of Social and Economic Context." *Kennedy Institute of Ethics Journal* 23(4): 355–79.

Fisher, Jill A. 2020. *Adverse Events: Race, Inequality and the Testing of New Pharmaceuticals*. New York: New York University Press.

Fisher, Max, Amanda Taub, and Dalia Martínez. 2018. "Losing Faith in the State, Some Mexican Towns Quietly Break Away." *New York Times*, January 7, A1.

Flores, Edward. 2014. *God's Gangs: Barrio Ministry, Masculinity, and Gang Recovery*. New York: New York University Press.

Folayan, Morenike Oluwatoyin, Bridget Haire, Kristin Peterson, and Aminu Yakubu et al. 2019. "Criminalisation and 'Reckless' Ebola Transmission: Theorizing Ethical Obligations to Seek Care." In *Socio-cultural Dimensions of Emerging Infectious Diseases in Africa: An Indigenous Response to Deadly Epidemics*, edited by Godfrey B. Tangwa, Akin Abayomi, Samuel J. Ujewe, and Nchangwi Syntia Munung, 229–42. Cham, Switzerland: Springer.

Ford, Andrea. 2019. "Triple Toxicity." *Fieldsights*. https://culanth.org/fieldsights/triple-toxicity.

Freeman, Carla. 2014. *Entrepreneurial Selves: Neoliberal Respectability and the Making of a Caribbean Middle Class*. Durham, NC: Duke University Press.

Fuentes, Agustín. 2019. "Holobionts, Multispecies Ecologies, and the Biopolitics of Care: Emerging Landscapes of Praxis in a Medical Anthropology of the Anthropocene." *Medical Anthropology Quarterly* 33(1): 156–62.

Fuentes, Agustín, Rebecca Rogers Ackermann, Sheela Athreya, and Deborah Bolnick et al. 2019. "AAPA Statement on Race and Racism." *American Journal of Physical Anthropology* 169(3): 400–402.

Fuentes, Mario Luis. 2013. "Marginación: Una pobreza desigual en México." *Excelsior*, August 13. https://www.excelsior.com.mx/nacional/2013/08/13/913401.

Galeana, Patricia, and Patricia Vargas Becerra. 2015. *Géneros asimétricos: Representaciones y percepciones del imaginario colectivo*. Encuesta Nacional de Género. Mexico City: Universidad Nacional Autónoma de México.

Gamlin, Jennie B., and Sarah J. Hawkes. 2017. "Masculinities on the Continuum of Structural Violence: The Case of Mexico's Homicide Epidemic." *Social Politics: International Studies in Gender, State and Society* 25(1): 50–71.

Garrard-Burnett, Virginia, and David Stoll, Eds. 1993. *Rethinking Protestantism in Latin America*. Philadelphia: Temple University Press.

Gaut, Berys. 1995. "Rawls and the Claims of Liberal Legitimacy." *Philosophical Papers* 24(1): 1–22.

Geissler, P. Wenzel. 2011. "Studying Trial Communities: Anthropological and Historical Inquiries into Ethos, Politics and Economy of Medical Research in Africa." In *Evidence, Ethos and Experiment: The Anthropology and History of Medical Research in Africa*, edited by P. Wenzel Geissler and Catherine Molyneux, 1–28. New York: Berghahn.

Geissler, P. Wenzel. 2013. "Public Secrets in Public Health: Knowing Not to Know while Making Scientific Knowledge." *American Ethnologist* 40(1): 13–34.

Geissler, P. Wenzel, ed. 2015. *Para-states and Medical Science: Making African Global Health*. Durham, NC: Duke University Press.

Geissler, P. Wenzel, Ann Kelly, Babatunde Imoukhuede, and Robert Pool. 2008. "He Is Now Like a Brother, I Can Even Give Him Some Blood'—Relational Ethics and Material Exchanges in a Malaria Vaccine 'Trial Community' in the Gambia." *Social Science and Medicine* 67(5): 696–707.

Geissler, P. Wenzel, and Catherine Molyneux. 2011. *Evidence, Ethos and Experiment: The Anthropology and History of Medical Research in Africa*. New York: Berghahn.

Genus, Sandalia. 2018. "Building a Legacy? Ambivalent Impacts of a Malaria Vaccine Clinical Trial." *Journal of Material Culture* 23(4): 413–25.

Gerrets, Rene. 2015. "International Health and the Proliferation of 'Partnerships': (Un)intended Boost for State Institutions in Tanzania?" In *Para-States and Medical Science: Making African Global Health*, edited by P. Wenzel Geissler, 179–206. Durham, NC: Duke University Press.

Gerrits, Trudie. 2018. "Gender Dynamics, Sensitive Issues and Ethical Considerations in 'Joint Interviews' with Dutch Couples Undergoing Fertility Treatments." *Salute e Società* 18: 11–28.

Gilbertson, Adam, Elizabeth Poole Kelly, Stuart Rennie, and Gail Henderson et al. 2018. "Indirect Benefits in HIV Cure Clinical Research: A Qualitative Analysis." *AIDS Research and Human Retroviruses* 35(1): 100–107.

Gillison, Maura L., Anil K. Chaturvedi, and Douglas R. Lowy. 2008. "HPV Prophylactic Vaccines and the Potential Prevention of Noncervical Cancers in Both Men and Women." *Cancer* 113(S10): 3036–46.

Giuliano, Anna R., Eduardo Lazcano-Ponce, Luisa L. Villa, and Roberto Flores et al. 2008. "The Human Papillomavirus Infection in Men Study: Human Papillomavirus Prevalence and Type Distribution among Men Residing in Brazil, Mexico, and the United States." *Cancer Epidemiology Biomarkers and Prevention* 17(8): 2036–43.

Giuliano, Anna R., Eduardo Lazcano, Luisa L. Villa, and Jorge Salmeron et al. 2006. "Natural History of HPV Infection in Men: The HIM study." *AACR Meeting Abstracts* 2006(3): B215.

González-López, Gloria. 2005. *Erotic Journeys: Mexican Immigrants and Their Sex Lives.* Berkeley: University of California Press.

González-López, Gloria. 2015. *Family Secrets: Stories of Incest and Sexual Violence in Mexico.* New York: New York University Press.

González-Santos, Sandra P. 2020. *A Portrait of Assisted Reproduction in Mexico: Scientific, Political, and Cultural Interactions.* Cham, Switzerland: Palgrave Macmillan.

Goodman, Alan H, and Thomas Leland Leatherman. 2010. *Building a New Biocultural Synthesis: Political-Economic Perspectives on Human Biology.* Ann Arbor: University of Michigan Press.

Govindrajan, Radhika. 2018. *Animal Intimacies: Interspecies Relatedness in India's Central Himalayas.* Chicago: University of Chicago Press.

Gravlee, Clarence C. 2009. "How Race Becomes Biology: Embodiment of Social Inequality." *American Journal of Physical Anthropology* 139(1): 47–57.

Gregg, Jessica L. 2003. *Virtually Virgins: Sexual Strategies and Cervical Cancer in Recife, Brazil.* Stanford, CA: Stanford University Press.

Gutiérrez Chong, Natividad. 2017. "Violencia obstétrica en madres indígenas: Un caso de racismo." In *¡A toda madre! Una mirada multidisciplinaria a las maternidades en México*, edited by Abril Saldaña-Tejeda, Lilia Venegas Aguilera, and Tine Davids, 41–70. Mexico City: Científica.

Gutmann, Matthew C. 1996. *The Meanings of Macho: Being a Man in Mexico City.* Berkeley: University of California Press.

Gutmann, Matthew C. 2007. *Fixing Men: Sex, Birth Control, and AIDS in Mexico.* Berkeley: University of California Press.

Haenssgen, Marco J., Nutcha Charoenboon, and Yuzana Khine Zaw. 2018. "Is It Time to Give Social Research a Voice to Tackle Antimicrobial Resistance?" *Journal of Antimicrobial Chemotherapy* 73(4): 1112–13.

Hale, Kathryn Law. 2017. "Family Life and Social Medicine: Discourses and Discontents Surrounding Puebla's Psychiatric Care." *Culture, Medicine, and Psychiatry* 41(4): 499–540.

Hammar, Lawrence. 2007. "The Many Sexes of Risk: Gender, Disease, and Identity in the Asia-Pacific Region and Elsewhere." *Reviews in Anthropology* 36(4): 335–56.

Hammar, Lawrence. 2010. *Sin, Sex and Stigma: A Pacific Response to HIV and AIDS.* Wantage, UK: Sean Kingston.

Haney, Charlotte. 2012. "Imperiled Femininity: The Dismembering of Citizenship in Northern Mexico." *Journal of Latin American and Caribbean Anthropology* 17(2): 238–56.

Haraway, Donna J. 1988. "Situated Knowledges: The Science Question in Feminism and the Privilege of Partial Perspective." *Feminist Studies* 14: 575–99.

Haraway, Donna J. 2008. *When Species Meet*. Minneapolis: University of Minnesota Press.

Hardin, Jessica A. 2013. "Fasting for Health, Fasting for God: Samoan Evangelical Christian Responses to Obesity and Chronic Disease." In *Reconstructing Obesity: The Meaning of Measures and the Measure of Meanings*, edited by Megan B. McCullough and Jessica A. Hardin, 107–28. New York: Berghahn.

Heath, Melanie. 2003. "Soft-Boiled Masculinity: Renegotiating Gender and Racial Ideologies in the Promise Keepers Movement." *Gender and Society* 17(3): 423–44.

Herdt, Gilbert, and Shirley Lindenbaum, eds. 1992. *The Time of AIDS*. Newbury Park, CA: Sage.

Heron, Adom Philogene. 2019. "Being Said/Seen to Care: Masculine Silences and Emerging Visibilities of Intimate Fatherhood in Dominica, Lesser Antilles." In *Discourses from Latin America and the Caribbean: Current Concepts and Challenges*, edited by Eleonora Esposito, Carolina Pérez-Arredondo, and José Manuel Ferreiro, 267–98. Cham, Switzerland: Springer.

Hind, Emily. 2017. "Gente Decente and Civil Rights: From Suffrage to Divorce and Privileges in Between." In *Modern Mexican Culture: Critical Foundations*, edited by Stuart A. Day, 184–202. Tucson: University of Arizona Press.

Hirsch, Jennifer S. 2003. *A Courtship after Marriage: Sexuality and Love in Mexican Transnational Families*. Berkeley: University of California Press.

Hirsch, Jennifer S. 2008. "Catholics Using Contraceptives: Religion, Family Planning, and Interpretive Agency in Rural Mexico." *Studies in Family Planning* 39(2): 93–104.

Hirsch, Jennifer S., Jennifer Higgins, Margaret E. Bentley, and Constance A. Nathanson. 2002. "The Social Constructions of Sexuality: Marital Infidelity and Sexually Transmitted Disease—HIV Risk in a Mexican Migrant Community." *American Journal of Public Health* 92(8): 1227–37.

Hirsch, Jennifer S., Sergio Meneses, Brenda Thompson, and Mirka Negroni et al. 2007. "The Inevitability of Infidelity: Sexual Reputation, Social Geographies, and Marital HIV Risk in Rural Mexico." *American Journal of Public Health* 97(6): 986–96.

Hirsch, Jennifer S., and Constance A. Nathanson. 2001. "Some Traditional Methods Are More Modern than Others: Rhythm, Withdrawal and the Changing Meanings of Sexual Intimacy in Mexican Companionate Marriage." *Culture, Health and Sexuality* 3(4): 413–28.

Hirsch, Jennifer S., Holly Wardlow, Daniel Jordan Smith, and Harriet M. Phinney et al., eds. 2009. *The Secret: Love, Marriage, and HIV*. Nashville, TN: Vanderbilt University Press.

Hoffmann, Elizabeth A. 2007. "Open-ended Interviews, Power, and Emotional Labor." *Journal of Contemporary Ethnography* 36(3): 318–46.

Hoffmaster, Barry. 2018. "From Applied Ethics to Empirical Ethics to Contextual Ethics." *Bioethics* 32(2): 119–25.

Howes-Mischel, Rebecca. 2016. "'With This You Can Meet Your Baby': Fetal Personhood and Audible Heartbeats in Oaxacan Public Health." *Medical Anthropology Quarterly* 30(2): 186–202.

Hughes, Shana D., Nicolas Sheon, Erin V. W. Andrew, and Stephanie E. Cohen et al. 2018. "Body/Selves and Beyond: Men's Narratives of Sexual Behavior on PrEP." *Medical Anthropology* 37(5): 387–400.

Hunt, Linda M. 1998. "Moral Reasoning and the Meaning of Cancer: Causal Explanations of Oncologists and Patients in Southern Mexico." *Medical Anthropology Quarterly* 12(3): 298–318.

Hunt, Nancy Rose. 1999. *A Colonial Lexicon: Of Birth Ritual, Medicalization, and Mobility in the Congo*. Durham, NC: Duke University Press.

Hunter, Mark. 2010. *Love in the Time of AIDS: Inequality, Gender, and Rights in South Africa*. Bloomington: Indiana University Press.

Inhorn, Marcia C. 2003. *Local Babies, Global Science: Gender, Religion and In Vitro Fertilization in Egypt*. New York: Routledge.

Inhorn, Marcia C. 2012. *The New Arab Man: Emergent Masculinities, Technologies, and Islam in the Middle East*. Princeton, NJ: Princeton University Press.

Instituto Nacional de Estadística y Geografía (INEGI). 2009. "Geográfica." http://www .inegi.org.mx/inegi/default.aspx?s=geo.

Instituto Nacional de Estadística y Geografía (INEGI). 2011. "Panorama de las religiones en México 2010." *Aguascalientes*. http://www.inegi.org.mx/prod_serv /contenidos/espanol/bvinegi/productos/censos/poblacion/2010/panora_religion /religiones_2010.pdf.

Jackson, Michael. 1998. *Minima Ethnographica: Intersubjectivity and the Anthropological Project*. Chicago: University of Chicago Press.

Janzen, Rebecca. 2015. *The National Body in Mexican Literature: Collective Challenges to Biopolitical Control*. Cham, Switzerland: Palgrave Macmillan.

Jennings, Bruce. 2016. "Reconceptualizing Autonomy: A Relational Turn in Bioethics." *Hastings Center Report* 46(3): 11–16.

Jordan, Sara R., and Phillip W. Gray. 2018. "Clarifying the Concept of the 'Social' in Risk Assessments for Human Subjects Research." *Accountability in Research* 25(1): 1–20.

Joseph, Gilbert M., Anne Rubenstein, and Eric Zolov. 2001. "Assembling the Fragments: Writing a Cultural History of Mexico since 1940." In *Fragments of a Golden Age: The Politics of Culture in Mexico since 1940*, edited by Gilbert M. Joseph, Anne Rubenstein, and Eric Zolov, 3–22. Durham, NC: Duke University Press.

Kahn, Susan Martha. 2000. *Reproducing Jews: A Cultural Account of Assisted Conception in Israel*. Durham, NC: Duke University Press.

Kamat, Vinay R. 2014. "Fast, Cheap, and Out of Control? Speculations and Ethical Concerns in the Conduct of Outsourced Clinical Trials in India." *Social Science and Medicine* 104: 48–55.

Kelly-Hanku, Angela, Peter Aggleton, and Patti Shih. 2014. "'We Call It a Virus but I Want to Say It's the Devil Inside': Redemption, Moral Reform and Relationships with God among People Living with HIV in Papua New Guinea." *Social Science and Medicine* 119: 106–13.

Kelly, Patty. 2008. *Lydia's Open Door: Inside Mexico's Most Modern Brothel*. Berkeley: University of California Press.

Kingfisher, Catherine, and Jeff Maskovsky. 2008. "Introduction: The Limits of Neoliberalism." *Critique of Anthropology* 28(2): 115–26.

Kingori, Patricia. 2013. "Experiencing Everyday Ethics in Context: Frontline Data Collectors' Perspectives and Practices of Bioethics." *Social Science and Medicine* 98: 361–70.

Kleinman, Arthur. 1980. *Patients and Healers in the Context of Culture*. Berkeley: University of California Press.

Kleinman, Arthur. 1995. "Anthropology of Bioethics." In *Writing at the Margin: Discourse between Anthropology and Medicine*, edited by Arthur Kleinman, 41–67. Berkeley: University of California Press.

Kleinman, Arthur, and Peter Benson. 2006. "Anthropology in the Clinic: The Problem of Cultural Competency and How to Fix It." *PLOS Medicine* 3(10): e294.

Knight, Alan. 1990. "Racism, Revolution, and Indigenismo: Mexico, 1910–1940." In *The Idea of Race in Latin America, 1870–1940*, edited by Richard Graham, 71–113. Austin: University of Texas Press.

Knight, Alan. 1992. "The Peculiarities of Mexican History: Mexico Compared to Latin America, 1821–1992." *Journal of Latin American Studies* 24: 99–144.

Knight, Alan. 2012. "Narco-violence and the State in Modern Mexico." In *Violence, Coercion, and State-making in Twentieth-Century Mexico: The Other Half of the Centaur*, edited by Wil G. Pansters, 115–34. Stanford, CA: Stanford University Press.

Kremer-Sadlik, Tamar. 2019. "Ordinary Ethics and Reflexivity in Mundane Family Interactions." *Ethos* 47(2): 190–210.

Krieger, Nancy. 2012. "Methods for the Scientific Study of Discrimination and Health: An Ecosocial Approach." *American Journal of Public Health* 102(5): 936–44.

La Redacción. 2016. "Más de 35 mil personas en la marcha por la paz." La Unión de Morelos. http://www.launion.com.mx/morelos/avances/noticias/89753-mas-de-35-mil-personas-en-la-marcha-por-la-paz.html

Leach, Melissa, and James Fairhead. 2011. "Being 'with Medical Research Council': Infant Care and the Social Meanings of Cohort Membership in Gambia's Plural Therapeutic Landscapes." In *Evidence, Ethos and Experiment: The Anthropology and History of Medical Research in Africa*, edited by P. Wenzel Geissler and Catherine Molyneux, 77–98. New York: Berghahn.

León-Maldonado, Leith, Emily Wentzell, Brandon Brown, and Betania Allen-Leigh et al. 2016. "Perceptions and Experiences of Human Papillomavirus (HPV) Infection and Testing among Low-Income Mexican Women." *PLOS One* 11(5): e0153367.

Lester, Rebecca J. 2007. "Critical Therapeutics: Cultural Politics and Clinical Reality in Two Eating Disorder Treatment Centers." *Medical Anthropology Quarterly* 21(4): 369–87.

LeVine, Sarah. 1993. *Dolor y Alegría: Women and Social Change in Urban Mexico*. Madison: University of Wisconsin Press.

Linde, Charlotte. 1993. *Life Stories: The Creation of Coherence*. New York: Oxford University Press.

Lock, Margaret. 1993. *Encounters with Aging: Mythologies of Menopause in Japan and North America*. Berkeley: University of California Press.

Lock, Margaret, and Patricia Kaufert. 2001. "Menopause, Local Biologies, and Cultures of Aging." *American Journal of Human Biology* 13(4): 494–504.

Lock, Margaret, and Vinh-Kim Nguyen. 2018. *An Anthropology of Biomedicine.* New York: John Wiley and Sons.

Lomnitz-Adler, Claudio. 2001. *Deep Mexico, Silent Mexico: An Anthropology of Nationalism.* Minneapolis: University of Minnesota Press.

López-Beltrán, Carlos, and Vivette García Deister. 2013. "Aproximaciones científicas al mestizo mexicano." *História, Ciências Saúde–Manguinhos* 20(2): 391–410.

Lopez, Christian. 2015. "Trabajadores del IMSS protestan contra privatización. Diario de México," July 31. http://www.diariodemexico.com.mx/trabajadores-del-imss-protestan-contra-privatizacion.

Lorimer, Jamie. 2019. "Hookworms Make Us Human: The Microbiome, Eco-immunology, and a Probiotic Turn in Western Health Care." *Medical Anthropology Quarterly* 33(1): 60–79.

Love, David. 2015. "Mexico Officially Recognizes 1.38 Million Afro-Mexicans in the National Census, as Black People Fight against Racism and Invisibility throughout Latin America." *Atlanta Blackstar*, December 14. https://atlantablackstar.com/2015/12/14/mexico-officially-recognizes-1-38-million-afro-mexicans-in-the-national-census-as-black-people-fight-against-racism-and-invisibility-throughout-latin-america.

Luna, Sarah. 2018. "Affective Atmospheres of Terror on the Mexico-U.S. Border: Rumors of Violence in Reynosa's Prostitution Zone." *Cultural Anthropology* 33(1): 58–84.

Lupton, Deborah. 2016. "The Diverse Domains of Quantified Selves: Self-tracking Modes and Dataveillance." *Economy and Society* 45(1): 101–22.

Lupton, Deborah. 2019. "The Thing-Power of the Human-App Health Assemblage: Thinking with Vital Materialism." *Social Theory and Health* 17(2): 125–39.

Lyon, David, Kirstie Ball, and Kevin D. Haggerty, Eds. 2012. *Routledge Handbook of Surveillance Studies.* New York: Routledge.

Ma, Zhiying. 2019. "Family." *Somatosphere.* http://somatosphere.net/2019/01/family.html.

MacLeod, Dag. 2004. *Downsizing the State: Privatization and the Limits of Neoliberal Reform in Mexico.* University Park, PA: Penn State University Press.

Macleod, Morna, and Natalia De Marinis. 2018. *Resisting Violence: Emotional Communities in Latin America.* Cham, Switzerland: Palgrave Macmillan.

Magny, Caroline. 2009. "Cuando ya no se puede tomar trago ni chacchar coca: El caso de los conversos 'protestantes' en los Andes centrales peruanos." *Anthropology of Food* (online) S6: n.p.

Manrique, Linnete. 2016. "Dreaming of a Cosmic Race: José Vasconcelos and the Politics of Race in Mexico, 1920s–1930s." *Cogent Arts and Humanities* 3(1): 1218316.

Manrique, Linnete. 2017. "Making the Nation: The Myth of Mestizajes." *Anthropology* 5(186): n.p.

Marshall, Patricia, David C. Thomasma, and Jurrit Bergsma. 1994. "Intercultural Reasoning: The Challenge for International Bioethics." *Cambridge Quarterly of Healthcare Ethics* 3(3): 321–28.

Mason, Katherine A. 2018. "Quantitative Care: Caring for the Aggregate in U.S. Academic Population Health Sciences." *American Ethnologist* 45(2): 201–13.

Matsuura, Hiroaki. 2013. "The Effect of a Constitutional Right to Health on Population Health in 157 Countries, 1970–2007: The Role of Democratic Governance." Working Paper no. 106. Program on the Global Demography of Aging, Harvard University, Cambridge, MA.

McGranahan, Carole. 2018. "Ethnography beyond Method: The Importance of an Ethnographic Sensibility." *Sites* 15(1): 1–10.

McKee Irwin, Robert. 2003. *Mexican Masculinities*. Minneapolis: University of Minnesota Press.

Melero, Pilar. 2015. *Mythological Constructs of Mexican Femininity*. New York: Palgrave Macmillan.

Melgar Bao, Ricardo. 2005. "Poder y simbolismo escultórico en Cuernavaca." In *IV Coloquio Paul Kirchhoff: Las expresiones del poder, homenaje al Doctor Claudio Esteva Fabregat*, edited by Rafael Pérez-Taylor, 193–201. Mexico City: Instituto de Investigaciones Antropológicas, Universidad Nacional Autónoma de México.

Melhuus, Marit. 1996. "Power, Value and the Ambiguous Meanings of Gender." In *Machos, Mistresses, Madonnas: Contesting the Power of Latin American Gender Imagery*, edited by Marit Melhuus and Kristi Anne Stølen, 230–59. London: Verso.

Melhuus, Marit. 1998. "Configuring Gender: Male and Female in Mexican Heterosexual and Homosexual Relations." *Ethnos* 63(3): 353–82.

Meloni, Maurizio. 2014. "Remaking Local Biologies in an Epigenetic Time." *Somatosphere*. http://somatosphere.net/2014/remaking-local-biologies-in-an-epigenetic-time.html.

Meloni, Maurizio, John Cromby, Des Fitzgerald, and Stephanie Lloyd. 2018. "Introducing the New Biosocial Landscape." In *The Palgrave Handbook of Biology and Society*, edited by Maurizio Meloni, John Cromby, Des Fitzgerald and Stephanie Lloyd, 1–22. Cham, Switzerland: Springer.

Metzl, Jonathan M., and Helena Hansen. 2014. "Structural Competency: Theorizing a New Medical Engagement with Stigma and Inequality." *Social Science and Medicine* 103: 126–33.

Meynell, Letitia, and Kirstin Borgerson. 2020. "Susan Sherwin: Shaping a More Just Bioethics." *International Journal of Feminist Approaches to Bioethics* 13(2): 1–8.

Mezo Gonzalez, Juan Carlos. 2018. "Macho Tips: The Erotics of the Mexican Body in a Gay Magazine." NOTCHES: *(Re)marks on the History of Sexuality*. http://notchesblog.com/2018/09/18/macho-tips-the-erotics-of-the-mexican-body-in-a-gay-magazine.

Miranda, Justino. 2012. "Cinco cárteles se disputan Morelos." *El Universal*, September 22. http://www.eluniversal.com.mx/notas/871981.html.

Misra, Amalendu. 2012. "My Space/Mi Espacio: Evangelical Christianity and Identity Politics in Mexico." *Bulletin of Latin American Research* 31(1): 65–79.

Molyneux, C. S., N. Peshu, and K. Marsh. 2005. "Trust and Informed Consent: Insights from Community Members on the Kenyan Coast." *Social Science and Medicine* 61(7): 1463–73.

Molyneux, Sassy, and P. Wenzel Geissler. 2008. "Ethics and the Ethnography of Medical Research in Africa." *Social Science and Medicine* 67(5): 685–95.

Montgomery, Catherine M. 2012. "Making Prevention Public: The Co-production of Gender and Technology in HIV Prevention Research." *Social Studies of Science* 42(6): 922–44.

Montoya, Michael J. 2011. *Making the Mexican Diabetic: Race, Science and the Genetics of Inequality.* Berkeley: University of California Press.

Morales-Campos, Daisy Y., S. A. Snipes, E. K. Villarreal, and L. C. Crocker et al. 2018. "Cervical Cancer, Human Papillomavirus (HPV), and HPV Vaccination: Exploring Gendered Perspectives, Knowledge, Attitudes, and Cultural Taboos among Mexican American Adults." *Ethnicity and Health* 26(2): 1–19.

Moreno Figueroa, Mónica G. 2010. "Distributed Intensities: Whiteness, Mestizaje and the Logics of Mexican Racism." *Ethnicities* 10(3): 387–401.

Moreno Figueroa, Mónica G., and Emiko Saldívar Tanaka. 2015. "'We Are Not Racists, We Are Mexicans': Privilege, Nationalism and Post-Race Ideology in Mexico." *Critical Sociology* 42(4–5): 515–33.

Moreno, Pedro, Silvia Tamez, and Claudia Ortiz. 2009. *Social Security in Mexico.* Solidarity Center. http://www.solidaritycenter.org/files/WorkingMexicoChapter10.pdf.

Morgan, Lynn M. 1996. "Fetal Relationality in Feminist Philosophy: An Anthropological Critique." *Hypatia* 11(3): 47–70.

Morris, Norma, and Brian Bàlmer. 2006. "Volunteer Human Subjects' Understandings of Their Participation in a Biomedical Research Experiment." *Social Science and Medicine* 62(4): 998–1008.

Morris, Rosalind C. 1995. "All Made Up: Performance Theory and the New Anthropology of Sex and Gender." *Annual Review of Anthropology* 24: 567–92.

Mortensen, Gitte, and Helle Larsen. 2010. "The Quality of Life of Patients with Genital Warts: A Qualitative Study." *BMC Public Health* 10(1): 113.

Muller, Jessica H. 1994. "Anthropology, Bioethics, and Medicine: A Provocative Trilogy." *Medical Anthropology Quarterly* 8(4): 448–67.

Mullings, Leith. 2005. "Resistance and Resilience: The Sojourner Syndrome and the Social Context of Reproduction in Central Harlem." *Transforming Anthropology* 13(2): 79–91.

Nading, Alex M. 2013. "Humans, Animals, and Health: From Ecology to Entanglement." *Environment and Society* 4(1): 60–78.

Nading, Alex M. 2014. *Mosquito Trails: Ecology, Health, and the Politics of Entanglement.* Berkeley: University of California Press.

Napolitano, Valentina. 2002. *Migration, Mujercitas, and Medicine Men: Living in Urban Mexico.* Berkeley: University of California Press.

Napolitano, Valentina, and Gerardo Mora Flores. 2003. "Complementary Medicine: Cosmopolitan and Popular Knowledge, and Transcultural Translations—Cases from Urban Mexico." *Theory, Culture and Society* 20(4): 79–95.

Navarro, Carlos, and Miguel Leatham. 2004. "Pentecostal Adaptations in Rural and Urban México: An Anthropological Assessment." *Mexican Studies/Estudios Mexicanos* 20(1): 145–66.

Navarro-Hernández, Mariana, Nancy Reynoso-Noverón, and Amanda De la Piedra-Gómez. 2018. "Survey on the Use of Alternative and Complementary Medicine in Mexican Patients with Cancer in an Oncology Reference Center." *Gaceta Mexicana de Oncologia* 17: n.p.

Nehring, Daniel. 2011. "Negotiated Familism: Intimate Life and Individualization among Young Female Professionals from Mexico City." *Canadian Journal of Latin American and Caribbean Studies* 36(71): 165–96.

Nguyen, Vinh-Kim. 2009. "Government-by-Exception: Enrolment and Experimentality in Mass HIV Treatment Programmes in Africa." *Social Theory and Health* 7(3): 196–217.

Nguyen, Vinh-Kim. 2015. "Treating to Prevent HIV: Population Trials and Experimental Societies." In *Para-States and Medical Science: Making African Global Health*, edited by P. Wenzel Geissler, 47–77. Durham, NC: Duke University Press.

Nieves Delgado, Abigail. 2020. "The Face of the Mexican: Race, Nation, and Criminal Identification in Mexico." *American Anthropologist* 122(2): 356–68.

Niewöhner, Jörg, and Margaret Lock. 2018. "Situating Local Biologies: Anthropological Perspectives on Environment/Human Entanglements." *BioSocieties* 13(4): 681–97.

Notimex. 2014. "Investigan discriminaciones en clínica rural del IMSS." *El Economista*, March 23. http://eleconomista.com.mx/sociedad/2014/03/23/investigan-discriminaciones-clinica-rural-imss.

Obrist, Brigit. 2004. "Medicalization and Morality in a Weak State: Health, Hygiene and Water in Dar es Salaam, Tanzania." *Anthropology and Medicine* 11(1): 43–57.

Ong, Aihwa. 2006. *Neoliberalism as Exception: Mutations in Citizenship and Sovereignty*. Durham, NC: Duke University Press.

Ortiz-Ortega, Adriana, Ana Amuchástegui, and Marta Rivas. 1998. "Because 'They Were Born from Me': Negotiating Women's Rights in Mexico." In *Negotiating Women's Rights: Women's Perspectives across Countries and Cultures*, edited by Roz P. Petchesky and Karen Judd, 145–79. London: Zed.

Oudshoorn, Nelly. 2003. *The Male Pill: A Biography of a Technology in the Making*. Durham, NC: Duke University Press.

Padgett, Tim. 2011. "Why I Protest: Javier Sicilia of Mexico." *Time.com*, December 14. http://content.time.com/time/specials/packages/article/0,28804,2101745_2102138_2102238,00.html.

Padilla, Mark B., Jennifer S. Hirsch, Miguel Muñoz-Laboy, and Robert Sember et al., eds. 2007. *Love and Globalization: Transformations of Intimacy in the Contemporary World*. Nashville, TN: Vanderbilt University Press.

Pansters, Wil G., ed. 2012. *Violence, Coercion, and State-making in Twentieth-Century Mexico: The Other Half of the Centaur*. Stanford, CA: Stanford University Press.

Parikh, Shanti A. 2007. "The Political Economy of Marriage and HIV: The ABC Approach, 'Safe' Infidelity, and Managing Moral Risk in Uganda." *American Journal of Public Health* 97(7): 1198–1208.

Parikh, Shanti A. 2016. *Regulating Romance: Youth Love Letters, Moral Anxiety, and Intervention in Uganda's Time of AIDS*. Nashville, TN: Vanderbilt University Press.

Parker, Richard, Regina Maria Barbosa, and Peter Aggleton, eds. 2000. *Framing the Sexual Subject*. Berkeley: University of California Press.

Pastrana, Daniela. 2011. "Drug-Related Violence Closing in on Mexican Capital." Inter Press Service News Agency. http://www.ipsnews.net/2011/05/drug-related-violence -closing-in-on-mexican-capital.

Paz, Octavio. [1961] 1985. *The Labyrinth of Solitude and Other Writings*, translated by Lysander Kemp. New York: Grove Weidenfeld.

Peña González, Rodrigo. 2014. *Inseguridad en Cuernavaca: Botón de muestra de la violencia en Morelos*. Presented at the Woodrow Wilson Center, Coorporación Andina de Fomento, and Instituto Tecnológico de Monterrey's Workshop on Citizen Security in Mexico, Monterrey, Mexico, October 28.

Perez Lopez, Yvonne. 2017. "Mestizaje Ideology as Color-blind Racism: Students' Discourses of Colorism and Racism in Mexico." Ph.D. diss., Syracuse University, Syracuse, NY.

Peterson, Anna, Manuel Vásquez, and Philip Williams. 2001. "Introduction: Christianity and Social Change in the Shadow of Globalization." In *Christianity, Social Change, and Globalization in the Americas*, edited by Anna L. Peterson, Manuel A. Vásquez, and Philip J. Williams, 1–24. New Brunswick, NJ: Rutgers University Press.

Petryna, Adriana. 2003. *Life Exposed: Biological Citizens after Chernobyl*. Princeton, NJ: Princeton University Press.

Petryna, Adriana. 2005. "Ethical Variability: Drug Development and Globalizing Clinical Trials." *American Ethnologist* 32(2): 183–97.

Petryna, Adriana. 2009. *When Experiments Travel: Clinical Trials and the Global Search for Human Subjects*. Princeton, NJ: Princeton University Press.

Petryna, Adriana, and Karolina Follis. 2015. "Risks of Citizenship and Fault Lines of Survival." *Annual Review of Anthropology* 44: 401–17.

Pirinjian, Lori. 2019. "'Nation as Family' and the Causes of Gender-based Violence in Modern Armenia." Ph.D. diss., San Francisco State University.

Pirotta, M., L. Ung, A. Stein, and E. L. Conway et al. 2009. "The Psychosocial Burden of Human Papillomavirus Related Disease and Screening Interventions." *Sexually Transmitted Infections* 85(7): 508–13.

Pollak, Margaret. 2018. "Care in the Context of a Chronic Epidemic: Caring for Diabetes in Chicago's Native Community." *Medical Anthropology Quarterly* 32(2): 196–213.

Pomales, Tony O. 2013. "Men's Narratives of Vasectomy: Rearticulating Masculinity and Contraceptive Responsibility in San José, Costa Rica." *Medical Anthropology Quarterly* 27(1): 23–42.

Porter, Natalie. 2019. "Training Dogs to Feel Good: Embodying Well-being in Multispecies Relations." *Medical Anthropology Quarterly* 33(1): 101–19.

Povinelli, Elizabeth A. 2006. *The Empire of Love: Toward a Theory of Intimacy, Genealogy, and Carnality*. Durham, NC: Duke University Press.

Pritzker, Sonya E., and Whitney L. Duncan. 2019. "Technologies of the Social: Family Constellation Therapy and the Remodeling of Relational Selfhood in China and Mexico." *Culture, Medicine, and Psychiatry* 43(3): 468–95.

Quinlan, Jacklyn, Laurel N. Pearson, Christopher J. Clukay, and Miaisha M. Mitchell et al. 2016. "Genetic Loci and Novel Discrimination Measures Associated with Blood Pressure Variation in African Americans Living in Tallahassee." *PLOS One* 11(12): e0167700.

Rabinow, Paul. 1999. "Artificiality and Enlightenment: From Sociobiology to Biosociality." In *The Science Studies Reader*, edited by Mario Biagioli, 407–16. New York: Routledge.

Race, Kane. 2012. "'Frequent Sipping': Bottled Water, the Will to Health and the Subject of Hydration." *Body and Society* 18(3–4): 72–98.

Radin, Joanna. 2018. "Ethics in Human Biology: A Historical Perspective on Present Challenges." *Annual Review of Anthropology* 47(1): 263–78.

Rajtar, Małgorzata. 2018. "Relational Autonomy, Care, and Jehovah's Witnesses in Germany." *Bioethics* 32(3): 184–92.

Ramabu, Nankie M. 2019. "Whose Autonomy Is It? Botswana Socio-ethical Approach to the Consenting Process." *Developing World Bioethics*. Accessed September 29, 2020. https://doi.org/10.1111/dewb.12253.

Ramirez, Josué. 2009. *Against Machismo: Young Adult Voices in Mexico City*. New York: Berghahn.

Ramirez, Michelle, and Margaret Everett. 2018. "Imagining Christian Sex: Reproductive Governance and Modern Marriage in Oaxaca, Mexico." *American Anthropologist* 120(4): 684–96.

Rayzberg, Margarita S. 2019. "Fairness in the Field: The Ethics of Resource Allocation in Randomized Controlled Field Experiments." *Science, Technology, and Human Values* 44(3): 371–98.

Reihling, Hans. 2020. *Affective Health and Masculinities in South Africa: An Ethnography of (In)vulnerability*. New York: Routledge.

Reinharz, Shulamit, and Susan E. Chase. 2002. "Interviewing Women." In *Handbook of Interview Research: Context and Method*, edited by Jaber F. Gubrium and James A. Holstein, 221–38. Thousand Oaks, CA: Sage.

Reynolds, Joanna, Peter Mangesho, Martha M. Lemnge, and Lasse S. Vestergaard et al. 2013. "'. . . In the Project They Really Care for Us': Meaning and Experiences of Participating in a Clinical Study of First-Line Treatment for Malaria and HIV in Tanzanian Adults." *Global Public Health* 8(6): 670–84.

Roberts, Elizabeth F. S. 2006. "God's Laboratory: Religious Rationalities and Modernity in Ecuadorian In Vitro Fertilization." *Culture, Medicine and Psychiatry* 30:507–36.

Roberts, Elizabeth F. S. 2016. "When Nature/Culture Implodes: Feminist Anthropology and Biotechnology." In *Mapping Feminist Anthropology in the Twenty-first Century*, edited by Ellen Lewin and Leni M. Silverstein, 105–25. New Brunswick, NJ: Rutgers University Press.

Roberts, Elizabeth F. S., and Camilo Sanz. 2018. "Bioethnography: A How-To Guide for the Twenty-first Century." In *The Palgrave Handbook of Biology and Society*, edited by Maurizio Meloni, John Cromby, Des Fitzgerald, and Stephanie Lloyd, 749–75. London: Palgrave Macmillan.

Rose, Nikolas, and Carlos Novas. 2005. "Biological Citizenship." In *Global Assemblages: Technology, Politics and Ethics as Anthropological Problems*, edited by Aihwa Ong and Stephen J. Collier, 439–63. Malden, MA: Blackwell.

Roy, Rohan Deb. 2017. *Malarial Subjects: Empire, Medicine and Nonhumans in British India, 1820–1909*. Cambridge: Cambridge University Press.

Russo Garrido, Anahi. 2020. "Between Same-Sex Marriage, Convivencia, and Polyamory: A New Cartography of Queer Relationships in Mexico City." *Signs* 46(1): 127–49.

Saad-Filho, Alfredo, and Deborah Johnston. 2005. *Neoliberalism: A Critical Reader*. Chicago: University of Chicago Press.

Saldaña-Tejeda, Abril. 2018a. "Mitochondrial Mothers of a Fat Nation: Race, Gender and Epigenetics in Obesity Research on Mexican Mestizos." *BioSocieties* 13(2): 434–52.

Saldaña-Tejeda, Abril. 2018b. "Mothers' Experiences of Masculinity in the Context of Child Obesity in Mexico." *Women's Studies International Forum* 70:39–45.

Saldívar, Emiko. 2014. "'It's Not Race, It's Culture': Untangling Racial Politics in Mexico." *Latin American and Caribbean Ethnic Studies* 9(1): 89–108.

Sanders, Nichole. 2017. "Las mujeres, el trabajo y la maternidad durante el Milagro Mexicano (1940–1960). In *¡A toda madre! Una mirada multidisciplinaria a las maternidades en México*, edited by Abril Saldaña Tejeda, Lilia Venegas Aguilera, and Tine Davids, 309–36. Mexico City: Científica.

Sanders, Rachel. 2017. "Self-Tracking in the Digital Era: Biopower, Patriarchy, and the New Biometric Body Projects." *Body and Society* 23(1): 36–63.

Santoro, Pablo, and Carmen Romero-Bachiller. 2017. "Thinking (Bioeconomies) through Care: Patients' Engagement with the Bioeconomies of Parenting." In *Bioeconomies*, edited by Vincenzo Pavone and Joanna Goven, 279–302. Cham, Switzerland: Palgrave Macmillan.

Santos, Jose Leonardo. 2012. *Evangelicalism and Masculinity: Faith and Gender in El Salvador*. Lanham, MD: Lexington.

Sariola, Salla, and Bob Simpson. 2011. "Theorising the 'Human Subject' in Biomedical Research: International Clinical Trials and Bioethics Discourses in Contemporary Sri Lanka." *Social Science and Medicine* 73(4): 515–21.

Schensul, Stephen L., Abdelwahed Mekki-Berrada, Bonnie K. Nastasi, and Rajendra Singh et al. 2006. "Men's Extramarital Sex, Marital Relationships and Sexual Risk in Urban Poor Communities in India." *Journal of Urban Health* 83(4): 614–24.

Scheper-Hughes, Nancy, and Margaret M. Lock. 1987. "The Mindful Body: A Prolegomenon to Future Work in Medical Anthropology." *Medical Anthropology Quarterly* 1(1): 6–41.

Schneider, Suzanne D. 2010. *Mexican Community Health and the Politics of Health Reform*. Albuquerque: University of New Mexico Press.

Scott, Clare, Jan Walker, Peter White, and George Lewith. 2011. "Forging Convictions: The Effects of Active Participation in a Clinical Trial." *Social Science and Medicine* 72(12): 2041–48.

Seale-Feldman, Aidan. 2019. "Relational Affliction: Reconceptualizing 'Mass Hysteria.'" *Ethos* 47(3): 307–25.

Seale, Clive, Jonathan Charteris-Black, Carol Dumelow, and Louise Locock et al. 2008. The Effect of Joint Interviewing on the Performance of Gender. *Field Methods* 20(2): 107–28.

Seguridad, Justicia y Paz, Consejo Ciudadano para la Seguridad Pública y Justicia Penal A.C. 2012. *La violencia en los municipios de México 2012*. http://www

.seguridadjusticiaypaz.org.mx/sala-de-prensa/768-la-violencia-en-los-municipios
-de-mexico-2012.

Seguridad, Justicia y Paz, Consejo Ciudadano para la Seguridad Pública y Justicia
Penal A.C. 2015. *La violencia en los municipios y en las entidades federativas de México
2014.* http://www.seguridadjusticiaypaz.org.mx/biblioteca/download/6-prensa/205-la
-violencia-en-los-municipios-y-en-las-entidades-federativas-de-mexico-2014.

Selbekk, Anne Schanche, Peter J. Adams, and Hildegunn Sagvaag. 2018. "'A Problem like
This Is Not Owned by an Individual': Affected Family Members Negotiating Positions
in Alcohol and Other Drug Treatment." *Contemporary Drug Problems* 45(2): 146–62.

Shakuto, Shiori. 2019. "Postwork Intimacy: Negotiating Romantic Partnerships among
Japanese Retired Couples in Malaysia." *American Ethnologist* 46(3): 302–12.

Shaw, Rhonda M., ed. 2017. *Bioethics beyond Altruism.* Cham, Switzerland: Springer
International.

Sheikh, Zainab Afshan, and Anja M. B. Jensen. 2019. "Channeling Hope: An Ethnographic Study of How Research Encounters Become Meaningful for Families Suffering from Genetic Disease in Pakistan." *Social Science and Medicine* 228: 103–10.

Sherwin, Susan. 1998. "A Relational Approach to Autonomy in Health Care." In
The Politics of Women's Health: Exploring Agency and Autonomy, edited by Susan
Sherwin and Feminist Health Care Ethics Research Network, 19–47. Philadelphia:
Temple University Press.

Shim, Janet K. 2014. *Heart-sick: The Politics of Risk, Inequality, and Heart Disease.*
New York: New York University Press.

Shoveller, Jean A., et al. 2010. "'Not the Swab!': Young Men's Experiences with STI
Testing." *Sociology of Health and Illness* 32(1): 57–73.

Sierra, Justo. [1900] 1969. *The Political Evolution of the Mexican People*, translated by
Charles Ramsdell. Austin: University of Texas Press.

Simpson, Bob, Rekha Khatri, Deapica Ravindran, and Tharindi Udalagama. 2015.
"Pharmaceuticalisation and Ethical Review in South Asia: Issues of Scope and Authority for Practitioners and Policy Makers." *Social Science and Medicine* 131: 247–54.

Sims, Jennifer M. 2010. "A Brief Review of the Belmont Report." *Dimensions of Critical
Care Nursing* 29(4): 173–74.

Singer, Elyse Ona. 2017. "From Reproductive Rights to Responsibilization: Fashioning
Liberal Subjects in Mexico City's New Public Abortion Program." *Medical Anthropology Quarterly* 31(4): 445–63.

Singleton, Robyn, Jacqueline Carter, Tatianna Alencar, and Alicia Piñeirúa-Menéndez
et al. 2018. "Social Representations of Masculinity in Mexican Youth's Creative
Narratives." *Boyhood Studies* 11(1): 63–81.

Smith-Oka, Vania. 2012. "'They Don't Know Anything': How Medical Authority Con-
structs Perceptions of Reproductive Risk among Low-Income Mothers in Mexico."
In *Risk, Reproduction, and Narratives of Experience*, edited by Lauren Fordyce and
Amínata Maraesa, 103–22. Nashville, TN: Vanderbilt University Press.

Smith-Oka, Vania, and Megan K. Marshalla. 2019. "Crossing Bodily, Social, and Intimate Boundaries: How Class, Ethnic, and Gender Differences Are Reproduced in
Medical Training in Mexico." *American Anthropologist* 121(1): 113–25.

Smith, Daniel Jordan. 2004. "Youth, Sin and Sex in Nigeria: Christianity and HIV/AIDS-Related Beliefs and Behaviour among Rural-Urban Migrants." *Culture, Health and Sexuality* 6(5): 425–37.

Smith, Daniel Jordan. 2017. *To Be a Man Is Not a One-Day Job: Masculinity, Money, and Intimacy in Nigeria*. Chicago: University of Chicago Press.

Solomon, Harris. 2016. *Metabolic Living: Food, Fat, and the Absorption of Illness in India*. Durham, NC: Duke University Press.

Soto Laveaga, Gabriela. 2007. "'Let's Become Fewer': Soap Operas, Contraception, and Nationalizing the Mexican Family in an Overpopulated World." *Sexuality Research and Social Policy* 4(3): 19–33.

Springer, Kristen W., Jeanne Mager Stellman, and Rebecca M. Jordan-Young. 2012. "Beyond a Catalogue of Differences: A Theoretical Frame and Good Practice Guidelines for Researching Sex/Gender in Human Health. *Social Science and Medicine* 74(11): 1817–24.

Stadler, Jonathan, Hayley MacGregor, Eirik Saethre, and Sinead Delany-Moretlwe. 2018. "'Hold on' (Bambelela)! Lyrical Interpretations of Participation in an HIV Prevention Clinical Trial." *Culture, Health and Sexuality* 20(11): 1199–1213.

Stahler-Sholk, Richard. 2007. "Resisting Neoliberal Homogenization: The Zapatista Autonomy Movement." *Latin American Perspectives* 34(2): 48–63.

Stark, Laura. 2011. *Behind Closed Doors: IRBs and the Making of Ethical Research*. Chicago: University of Chicago Press.

Stepan, Nancy. 1991. *"The Hour of Eugenics": Race, Gender, and Nation in Latin America*. Ithaca, NY: Cornell University Press.

Stern, Alexandra M. 1999. "Responsible Mothers and Normal Children: Eugenics, Nationalism, and Welfare in Post-revolutionary Mexico, 1920–1940." *Journal of Historical Sociology* 12(4): 369–97.

Stern, Alexandra M. 2003. "From Mestizophilia to Biotypology: Racialization and Science in Mexico, 1920–1960." In *Race and Nation in Modern Latin America*, edited by Nancy P. Appelbaum, Anne S. Macpherson, and Karin Alejandra Rosemblatt, 187–210. Chapel Hill: University of North Carolina Press.

Stöckelová, Tereza, and Susanna Trnka. 2020. "Situating Biologies of Traditional Chinese Medicine in Central Europe." *Anthropology and Medicine* 27(1): 80–95.

Stoler, Ann Laura. 1989. "Making Empire Respectable: The Politics of Race and Sexual Morality in 20th Century Colonial Cultures." *American Ethnologist* 16(4): 634–60.

Street, Alice. 2012. "Seen by the State: Bureaucracy, Visibility and Governmentality in a Papua New Guinean Hospital." *Australian Journal of Anthropology* 23(1): 1–21.

Sue, Christina A. 2013. *Land of the Cosmic Race: Race Mixture, Racism, and Blackness in Mexico*. Oxford: Oxford University Press.

Sumich, Jason. 2016. "The Uncertainty of Prosperity: Dependence and the Politics of Middle-Class Privilege in Maputo." *Ethnos* 81(5): 821–41.

Sverdlin, Adina Radosh. 2017. "Bandas beyond Their 'Ethnographic Present': Neoliberalism and the Possibility of Meaning in Mexico City." *Journal of Extreme Anthropology* 1(3): 102–24.

Swallow, Julia, Anne Kerr, Choon Key Chekar, and Sarah Cunningham-Burley. 2020. "Accomplishing an Adaptive Clinical Trial for Cancer: Valuation Practices and Care Work across the Laboratory and the Clinic." *Social Science and Medicine* 252: 112949.

Thabethe, Siyabonga, Catherine Slack, Graham Lindegger, and Abigail Wilkinson et al. 2018. "'Why Don't You Go into Suburbs? Why Are You Targeting Us?': Trust and Mistrust in HIV Vaccine Trials in South Africa." *Journal of Empirical Research on Human Research Ethics* 13(5): 525–36.

Thayer, Zaneta M., and Christopher W. Kuzawa. 2011. "Biological Memories of Past Environments: Epigenetic Pathways to Health Disparities." *Epigenetics* 6(7): 798–803.

Tonantzin, Pedro. 2013. "El 30% de habitantes de Cuernavaca quiere emigrar por la inseguridad." *Excelsior en Linea*, April 13. http://www.excelsior.com.mx/nacional /2013/04/13/893626.

Torres-Poveda, Kirvis Janneth, Silvia Magali Cuadra-Hernández, Julieta Ivone Castro-Romero, and Vicente Madrid-Marina. 2011. "La política focalizada en el programa de vacunación contra el Virus del Papiloma Humano en México: Aspectos éticos." *Acta Bioethica* 17(1): 85–94.

Towghi, Fouzieyha. 2013. "The Biopolitics of Reproductive Technologies beyond the Clinic: Localizing HPV Vaccines in India." *Medical Anthropology* 32(4): 325–42.

Towghi, Fouzieyha, and Kalindi Vora. 2014. "Bodies, Markets, and the Experimental in South Asia." *Ethnos* 79(1): 1–18.

Tran, Allen L. 2018. "The Anxiety of Romantic Love in Ho Chi Minh City, Vietnam." *Journal of the Royal Anthropological Institute* 24(3): 512–31.

Trnka, Susanna, and Catherine Trundle. 2014. "Competing Responsibilities: Moving beyond Neoliberal Responsibilisation." *Anthropological Forum* 24(2): 136–53.

Tsing, Anna Lowenhaupt. 2015. *The Mushroom at the End of the World: On the Possibility of Life in Capitalist Ruins*. Princeton, NJ: Princeton University Press.

Turner, Edith. 2012. *Communitas: The Anthropology of Collective Joy*. New York: Palgrave Macmillan.

Turner, Victor. 1969. *The Ritual Process: Structure and Anti-structure*. New York: Routledge.

Twine, Rhian, Gillian Lewando Hundt, and Kathleen Kahn. 2017. "The 'Experimental Public' in Longitudinal Health Research: Views of Local Leaders and Service Providers in Rural South Africa." *Global Health Research and Policy* 2(1): 26.

Valdez, Natali. 2018. "The Redistribution of Reproductive Responsibility: On the Epigenetics of 'Environment' in Prenatal Interventions." *Medical Anthropology Quarterly* 32(3): 425–42.

Valdez, Natali. 2019. "Improvising Race: Clinical Trials and Racial Classification." *Medical Anthropology* 38(8): 635–50.

Valencia Triana, Sayak. 2012. "Capitalismo gore y necropolítica en México contemporáneo." *Relaciones Internacionales* 19: 83.

Van Anders, Sari M. 2013. "Beyond Masculinity: Testosterone, Gender/Sex, and Human Social Behavior in a Comparative Context." *Frontiers in Neuroendocrinology* 34(3): 198–210.

Van Klinken, Adriaan S. 2012. "Men in the Remaking: Conversion Narratives and Born-Again Masculinity in Zambia." *Journal of Religion in Africa* 42(3): 215–39.

Van Klinken, Adriaan S. 2013. *Transforming Masculinities in African Christianity: Gender Controversies in Times of AIDS*. Farnham, UK: Ashgate.

Vasconcelos, José. [1925] 1997. *The Cosmic Race: A Bilingual Edition*, translated by Didier T. Jaén. Baltimore: Johns Hopkins University Press.

Vaughan, Mary Kay. 1997. *Cultural Politics in Revolution: Teachers, Peasants, and Schools in Mexico, 1930–1940*. Tucson: University of Arizona Press.

Vaughan, Mary Kay, and Stephen E. Lewis, eds. 2006. *The Eagle and the Virgin: Nation and Cultural Revolution in Mexico, 1920–1940*. Durham, NC: Duke University Press.

Vaughn, Bobby. 2013. "Mexico Negro: From the Shadows of Nationalist Mestizaje to New Possibilities in Afro-Mexican Identity." *Journal of Pan African Studies* 6(1): 227–41.

Venables, Emilie, and Jonathan Stadler. 2012. "'The Study Has Taught Me to Be Supportive of Her': Empowering Women and Involving Men in Microbicide Research." *Culture, Health and Sexuality* 14(2): 181–94.

Vergara, Rosalía. 2016. "Privatización del IMSS pone en riesgo la salud de 71 millones de mexicanos." *Proceso.com*, December 16. http://www.proceso.com.mx/466658 /privatizacion-del-imss-pone-en-riesgo-la-salud-71-millones-mexicanos-pt.

Vieyra Bahena, Pedro. 2018. "La institucionalización fallida del individualismo en México de 1940 a 1970." *Sociológica (México)* 33(94): 269–301.

Viveiros de Castro, Eduardo. 1998. "Cosmological Deixis and Amerindian Perspectivism." *Journal of the Royal Anthropological Institute* 4(3): 469–88.

Wade, Peter. 2004. "Images of Latin American Mestizaje and the Politics of Comparison." *Bulletin of Latin American Research* 23(3): 355–66.

Waldby, Catherine. 2012. "Medicine: The Ethics of Care, the Subject of Experiment." *Body and Society* 18(3–4): 179–92.

Waller, Jo, Laura A. V. Marlow, and Jane Wardle. 2007. "The Association between Knowledge of HPV and Feelings of Stigma, Shame and Anxiety." *Sexually Transmitted Infections* 83(2): 155–59.

Walsh, Casey. 2004. "Eugenic Acculturation: Manuel Gamio, Migration Studies, and the Anthropology of Development in Mexico, 1910–1940." *Latin American Perspectives* 31(5): 118–45.

Wardlow, Holly, and Jennifer S. Hirsch, eds. 2006. *Modern Loves: The Anthropology of Romantic Courtship and Companionate Marriage*. Ann Arbor: University of Michigan Press.

Weaver, Lesley Jo. 2018. *Sugar and Tension: Diabetes and Gender in Modern India*. New Brunswick, NJ: Rutgers University Press.

Wegner, Mary Nell, Evelyn Landry, David Wilkinson, and Joanne Tzanis. 1998. "Men as Partners in Reproductive Health: From Issues to Action." *International Family Planning Perspectives* 24(1): 38–42.

Weiss, Gail. 1999. *Body Images: Embodiment as Intercorporeality*. New York: Routledge.

Wentzell, Emily A. 2013. *Maturing Masculinities: Aging, Chronic Illness, and Viagra in Mexico*. Durham, NC: Duke University Press.

Wentzell, Emily A., Yvonne N. Flores, Jorge Salmerón, and Roshan Bastani. 2016. "Factors Influencing Mexican Women's Decisions to Vaccinate Daughters against HPV in the United States and Mexico." *Family and Community Health* 39(4): 310–19.

Wentzell, Emily A., and Marcia C. Inhorn. 2014. "Reconceiving Masculinity and 'Men as Partners' for ICPD beyond 2014: Insights from a Mexican HPV Study." *Global Public Health* 9(6): 691–705.

Whyte, Susan Reynolds. 2011. "Writing Knowledge and Acknowledgement: Possibilities in Medical Research." In *Evidence, Ethos and Experiment: The Anthropology and History of Medical Research in Africa*, edited by P. Wenzel Geissler and Catherine Molyneux, 29–56. New York: Berghahn.

Wilkis, Ariel. 2015. "Thinking the Body: Durkheim, Mauss, Bourdieu: The Agreements and Disagreements of a Tradition." In *Thinking the Body as a Basis, Provocation, and Burden of Life*, edited by Gert Melville and Carlos Ruta, 33–44. Berlin: De Gruyter Oldenbourg.

Williams, David R., and Chiquita Collins. 1995. "U.S. Socioeconomic and Racial Differences in Health: Patterns and Explanations." *Annual Review of Sociology* 21(1): 349–86.

Wolters, Anna, Guido de Wert, Onna van Schayck, and Klasien Horstmann. 2014. "Constructing a Trial as a Personal Lifestyle Change Project: Participants' Experiences in a Clinical Study for Nicotine Vaccination." *Social Science and Medicine* 104: 116–23.

Wyss-van den Berg, Machteld, Bernhards Ogutu, Nelson K. Sewankambo, and Sonja Merten et al. 2020. "Communities and Clinical Trials: A Case Study from the RTS,S Malaria Vaccine Trials in Eastern Africa." *Journal of Empirical Research on Human Research Ethics.* 15(5): 465–77

Yarris, Kristin Elizabeth, and Carolyn Ponting. 2019. "Moral Matters: Schizophrenia and Masculinity in Mexico." *Ethos* 47(1): 35–53.

Yates-Doerr, Emily. 2017. "Where Is the Local? Partial Biologies, Ethnographic Sitings." *HAU: Journal of Ethnographic Theory* 7(2): 377–401.

Zabiliūtė, Emilija. 2020. "Ethics of Neighborly Intimacy among Community Health Activists in Delhi." *Medical Anthropology*. Accessed September 29, 2020. https://doi.org/10.1080/01459740.2020.1764550

Zhao, Jianhua. 2014. "Shame and Discipline: The Practice and Discourse of a 'Confucian Model' of Management in a Family Firm in China." *Critique of Anthropology* 34(2): 129–52.

Zolov, Eric. 1999. *Refried Elvis: The Rise of the Mexican Counterculture*. Berkeley: University of California Press.

Zuckerman, Molly K., and Debra L. Martin. 2016. "Introduction: The Development of Biocultural Perspectives in Anthropology." In *New Directions in Biocultural Anthropology*, edited by Molly K. Zuckerman and Debra L. Martin, 7–26. Hoboken, NJ: Wiley Blackwell.

individuality: Anglo-American ideas of, 7–8; and evangelical Christianity, 147; as focus of medical research, xi–xii, 3–4, 7–8, 84, 170–71; pressures to focus on, and collectivity, 163–66; refocusing object of inquiry beyond, 11, 159–60, 170–71; worldwide understandings of, 55, 108, 164, 173, 175, 179–80

inequalities, xi; mestizaje reinforces, 14, 16, 18; middle-class responses to, 54, 108; and research relationships, 8–9; United States as driver of, 32, 187

infidelity: and assignment of blame, 48, 50–51, 75–77; choice to refrain from, 38, 42, 76–77; discussion of with researcher, 183, 188; fears of, 53–54; health effects of, 47–48, 50, 140; STIs seen as sign of, 54, 71, 74–75, 142

insecurity crisis, Mexico, 1–2, 19, 88, 108, 119, 121, 126–28, 156; collectivist responses to, 165–66; in Cuernavaca, 22–25; and modeling of modernity, 125–28

Institutional Review Boards, 10, 177

Instituto Mexicano del Seguro Social (IMSS), 2, 24–25, 27, 83, 106, 147. *See also* Human Papillomavirus in Men (HIM) study

interrelatedness, 3–4, 10–11; of couples biology, 39, 41–42, 44, 51, 55, 61; cultural ideologies of, ix–x; and decision making, 2, 5, 8–9, 33, 43, 157, 160, 176, 179; despite bad behavior, 100–101; in evangelical churches, 148–49; familial, 97–98; and identity, 8, 9; social bodies as biological, 5, 79. *See also* collective biologies; couples biology; families

kinship, 9, 32, 163, 174, 188; *compradrazgo* (ritual), 29

Kleinman, Arthur, 175

Latin America: national racial ideologies, 14–15; violence in, 23–24

levels of scale, 11, 33–34, 83, 105; concentric, nested, 6, 157, 159–61; in evangelical Christianity, 145–46; masculinity as, 37. *See also* church; couples; families; nation; individual

life projects of research participants, 5–6, 28, 110, 121, 146, 162–63; moral projects, 2–3, 8, 14, 21

living for others, x, 2, 36, 111–12, 118, 163; in family roles, 84, 95, 97–98, 105; relational ethics approach, 176

local biologies, 4–5, 107, 164–65

local ideologies, 3–4, 33, 55–57, 151, 161, 163

Lock, Margaret, 4

Lopez Obrador, Andres Manuel, 127

Ma, Zhiying, 167

machismo, 33; and alcohol, 45–46, 99; attributed to conquistador ancestry, 18–19, 60, 62, 79–80; as bad for men's health, 45; blamed on regressive parenting, 40; Cristiano views of, 134–35, 139–44, 152; as cultural idea, 19, 63–64; emasculation, concerns about, 38–39; emerging Mexican ideas in opposition to, 37; in Guatemala, 88–89; as innate, belief in, 35–36, 38, 49–50, 51, 60–66, 79–80; life courses and relation to, 43, 50; men's rejection of, 35–45, 49–51, 61, 80; research participants on, 38–39, 49–51; seen as barrier, 20, 41

marginalized people, xi, 8, 165; damage from assignment to, 169–70; research participants, 3, 5–6, 9–10, 34, 158; as term for Indigenous and rural people, 14, 90

marriage: changing ideologies of, 31; egalitarian, 19–20; happiness of, 44, 49, 54, 74, 92–94, 103–4, 121, 124, 143, 145, 160; "healthy," 109; open, 68; same-sex, 20; "traditional," 20, 46–47, 54. *See also* companionate marriage

masculinity: anti-macho, 2, 35, 37, 38–42, 51; and care for others, 20–21; changing forms of, 37, 43; desired, 36–37; difference, assertion of, 49–51; effect of research participation on, 35–37; and explanatory models, 60; fidelity, commitment to, 38, 42; invulnerability, performance of, 39, 41, 78; men as penetrators, 39, 41, 43; modern/progressive, 2, 6, 9, 11, 21, 28, 39, 42–43, 60, 62, 93, 96, 112–13, 115; shame, gendered, 36, 39–40; transgression of traditional, 100–102; and vulnerability, 38–39, 50, 54. *See also* machismo; men mass hysteria/collective illness experience, 170

McGranahan, Carole, 31

medical research: Anglo-American ideas of, x–xi, 7–8, 162, 173; bioscientific, 170–75; clinical trials, 3, 5, 8–9, 26, 34, 157; context-specific approaches, 3–4, 59, 156, 168–69, 173–78; generalizability, 178; globalized, 3, 6–7, 10, 11, 34, 156, 158, 175–79; individual focus of, xi–xii, 3–4, 7–8, 84, 170–71; local, as lacking, 112–13; longitudinal and observational, 2–3, 5, 26, 58, 157–58, 178, 182–84; nonindividual bodies and understandings, ix, 11, 34, 151, 157–59, 163, 166–79; recruitment of participants, 7, 27–28, 65, 106, 174; as relational experience, 7–18; short-term, medically invasive, 5, 26; social consequences of, 7, 57, 72, 77, 80, 176–78, 186. *See also* research participation; social-science research; staff members

medicina popular, 136

men: guilt, feelings of, 48–49, 51, 65, 69–70, 72, 78, 100; rejection of machismo, 37, 43–45, 49–51, 61, 82–83; seen as carriers, 42, 60–61, 62, 63–67; seen as harmful to women, 57, 60, 62–66, 69, 73, 75, 79–80; seen as slow to mature, 21, 43, 45–46, 100. *See also* gender; machismo; masculinity

mental health issues, 165

mestizaje: ambivalence toward "Mexicanness," 17–18; "cosmic race" (*la raza cósmica*), 13, 14, 18, 125; Cristiano views of, 152–53; and gender norms, 13–14; and ideas of Mexican social body, 12–22; as identity, 12–22; and Indigenous peoples, xi, 12–16, 34; inequalities reinforced by, 14, 16, 18; marriage ideologies associated with, 20; "Mexican" as term for, 15, 17; as ongoing process, 15, 17–18; racially interrelated body, 3–4, 151; "regressive" tendencies, 18, 36, 62, 66, 89, 126

metaphors, used in explanatory models, 57–59, 109, 119–20

"Mexican," as term, 15, 17

Mexican national body, 4, 105, 106

Mexicanness. *See* mestizaje

Mexican Revolution (ca. 1910–20), 13, 19, 82

Mexico: citizen criticisms of, 23–25, 119–20, 126–29; as colonial enterprise, 165–66; constitutional mandate for healthcare, 13, 24, 57n1, 107–8, 161, 165; corruption in, 22–25, 113, 118–20, 127, 165; failure of to provide for citizens, 7, 16–18, 25, 108–11, 119–20, 126–29, 161, 164–65; genetics programs, 14–15; health campaigns, 13, 15, 16, 18, 54, 57, 107; insecurity crisis, 1–7, 19, 22–25, 88, 108, 119, 121, 126–28, 156, 165–66; medical system designed to improve nation, 16–17; nationalism, 12; presidential election, 2012, 119; privatization, 24–25, 107, 108, 164, 165; as "sick" culture, 119–21; single-party rule, 29; as "slippery state," 24, 33, 108–10, 121, 129; teachers' strikes, 120–21. *See also* Cuernavaca, Mexico; inequalities; nation

Mexico City, 22

middle class, 29, 107; assertion of through modern forms of intimacy, 54; capitalist tools used by, 158–59; definitions of, 3; *desarollo personal* (personal development), 43–44; family, views of, 29–30; identity projects of, 107, 128; intellectual interests, 38; modernity modeled by, 4, 6–7, 111–12, 158–59; parenting as marker of, 82, 96; trends influencing, 107

mixed methodologies, 169

modernity: communication as performance of, 73–74, 83; "cosmic race" (*la raza cósmica*), 13, 14, 18, 125; families different from unmodern others, 82, 88–90; indigeneity, move away from, 16–19, 79, 89, 106–7, 117, 163; machismo seen as barrier to, 20; and masculinity, 6, 9, 11, 21, 28, 39, 42–43, 60, 62, 93, 96, 112–13, 115; medical system designed around, 16–17; mixed expectations, 98; modeled by middle-class research participants, 4, 6–7, 111–12, 158–59; modeling at work, 117–18

Molyneux, Sassy, 11

Montgomery, Catherine, 9

Montoya, Michael, 174–75

Morelos State, 22–23, 108, 131

multilevel marketing companies, 132

muralist movement, 13

Napolitano, Valeria, 30, 136
narcoviolence, 1–2, 22, 37, 119–20, 165
nation, 13; "changing the culture," 36, 107, 114–21; "culture of ignorance," 16, 103, 107, 108, 110, 112, 115–18, 122, 124, 128–29; and "culture of prevention," 33, 108, 110, 113, 116–17; development, hopes for, 113; Mexican national body, 4, 105, 106; self-care as civic engagement, 106–11. *See also* collective biologies; Mexico
National Institutes of Health, 1–2, 26
neoliberal ideology, 108, 111, 113, 164, 179
Nepalese women, 170
nonindividual bodies and understandings, ix, 11, 34, 151, 157–59, 163, 166–79

Oaxaca State, 165
Oudshoorn, Nelly, 9

parenting, 38; anti-macho, 35–36, 51; as central to identity, 81, 83; companionate, 82–83; and drinking, 45–46; "goodness," discourse of, 82, 84–85, 94–97, 101–2, 105, 109, 160; incorporating HIM experiences into, 84–88; and research participation, 83–84; violence, fears of, 89, 96. *See also* families; fatherhood
participant observation, 31, 131, 186
personal development (*desarollo personal*), 43–44
personhood, 158–59, 183; Anglo-American ideas of, 7, 162, 166, 173; collective forms of, 133, 151, 156, 158, 162–68; Cristiano understanding of, 132–33, 135, 151; and ethics, 175–76; local cultural ideology of, 3–4; maternal-fetus collectivity, 168; "Mexican" as default "normal," 15; pious forms of, 135; racist and colonialist ideologies of, 173
Petryna, Adriana, 109
physicians, 16, 64, 184; and explanatory models, 58, 175; gender differences, and participant comfort, 40; as research participants, 39, 74, 83, 109; study procedures, 26–27, 39–40
police, as corrupt, 119, 127
political subcultures, 9
poor and marginalized populations, 5, 10, 90

portador, as term for male carrier, 64–67, 77–78, 160
privatization, 24–25, 107, 108, 164, 165
privileged categories, 12, 15–18, 27, 36, 106–7, 128, 165; Cristianos, 153; male, 134
public health: activism, 146–47; campaigns, 13, 15, 16, 18, 54, 57, 107; in Cuernavaca, 22–25; focus on women, 53, 56; implications for research, 7, 33–34, 156, 162, 172–73, 177–78, 183; modernity, discourses of, 107, 131; participant support of, 28, 42; practice, 177–78
Puebla, city of, 165
Puerto Rico, 170

race: as cultural ideology, 12, 15; as not scientifically valid, 12, 174
racial ideologies, 14–17, 51, 53, 135. *See also* mestizaje
relational ethics, 176
relationships: medical research as, 7–18; power-laden, 11. *See also* couples; couples biology; evangelical Christianity; families; interrelatedness; social body
religion. *See* church; evangelical Christians (Cristianos)
reproduction: assisted technologies, 82; value of, 81
"reproductive othering," 16
research participants: access to care, 10, 25, 28, 30, 39, 47, 57n1, 92, 99, 129, 136; as aspirational group, 106–7; and biological citizenship, 109–10; criticism of HIM study, 68, 148, 163; in health professions, 39–41; life projects of, 2–3, 5–6, 8, 14, 28–29, 110, 121, 146, 162–63; marginalized people as, 3, 5–6, 9–10, 34, 158; recruitment of, 7, 27–28, 65, 106; relationships with researchers, 8–9; resource-poor or marginalized, 3, 5, 6, 9–10, 34; supporting science, ix, 110, 111–13, 123; and "therapeutic misconception," 7–8, 10
research participation: as anti-macho act, 38–42; as citizenship practice, 7, 33, 110, 129; as entrepreneurial act, 10, 107–8, 126, 128, 132; and gender, 34; national change through, 36; and parenting, 83–84; racialized, 6; as way for men to be different, 49–51. *See also* medical research

respectable behavior, 8, 15, 18, 28, 54, 81, 104, 128

responsibility, 91, 95–96; companionate, 21, 28, 33, 37–38, 41–46, 50–51, 55, 66, 140; facilitated by testing, 42–43; personal, ideas about, 16, 108, 140, 173, 178–79

retirees, 110, 117, 124–25

"revolutionary" family, 14

Rivera, Diego, 13

Santos, Jose Leonardo, 134

Schneider, Susan, 108

science, supporting, ix, 110, 111–13, 123, 147

screening programs, 57, 63, 67, 77, 178

Seale-Feldman, Aidan, 170

self-care, 29–30, 38, 122–23; as civic engagement, 106–11; as collective care, 117, 144; and Cristianos, 135, 144; and families, 84–85, 87, 91–92, 97, 102, 104, 144; and masculinity, 21; and piety, 137

self-help, 43–44; and Cristianos, 132; military classes, 94, 111–12; personal growth groups, 114

sexual health, 2, 6, 42, 53–54, 102, 107; condom use, 68, 87, 97; education of children/teenagers, 24, 84, 92–93, 97–98, 104; gendered practices, 53–54; promotion of by research participants, 102, 115, 117; as shared, 31, 61–62, 71. See also health behavior

sexually transmitted infections (STIs): HPV as world's most common, 25, 56; stigma around, 54, 71, 181; testing for, 27, 36. See also human papillomavirus (HPV)

shame, gendered, 36, 39–40

Sicilia, Javier, 21

sickness metaphor, 119–21

situatedness, 168, 176

Slim, Carlos, 126

"slippery state," 24, 33, 108–10, 121, 129

smoking, and increased symptom risk, 58

social body, 4–6, 51, 161, 163–64; as biologically interrelated entities, 5, 79; and citizenship, 110; and discourse of "goodness," 82, 109–12, 120–21, 156, 159, 165, 183, 188; gender in, 18–22; mestizaje and ideas of Mexican, 12–22. See also collective biologies

social consequences of research, 7, 57, 72, 176–78, 186

social risks, 33, 54, 76–77, 142, 160, 182; and gendered ideas of biology, 77–80

social-science research, 3–8, 26, 34, 156–58, 162, 169–70, 176; ethnographic, ix, 31, 166, 168–69; methods, 168–69, 175, 181–86; as social forum, 99; as therapeutic for participants, 49. See also medical research

Somali region (Ethiopia), 11

staff members, 5, 10, 24; attempts to destigmatize HPV, 57; collective biologies recognized by, 174–75; educational efforts by, 57–59, 78, 107; interactions with participants, 26–27. See also medical research

stigma, 54, 71, 76–77; open secret model, 74; "sexual silence," 188; staff efforts to combat, 57

structural contexts, 5, 10–11, 90, 126, 156. See also cultural contexts

study-based communities, 9

study protocols, 3, 8, 171, 185

"subjects." See "human subjects"

surveillance medicine and self-surveillance, 178–79

testimonio, 132, 133, 148, 151, 154, 161

"therapeutic misconception," 7–8, 10

traditional healing practices, 30, 136

Trnka, Susanna, 164

Trundle, Catherine, 164

United States: research participant views of, 32, 187; Tuskegee syphilis study, 7

unit of analysis: collective biologies as, 167–68, 172; couples as, 5, 60, 157, 172, 182; ecosystem as, 172; families as, 167; individual as, 170–71

U.S.-Mexico borderlands, 174

vaccination: benefits of development, 85–86; dengue fever study, 113; programs, 57, 62

Vasconcelos, José, 13–14

violence: collective, 165; constraints on senior activities, 126–28; Cristiano responses to, 146, 149–50; in Latin America, 23–24; and machismo, 19, 21; narcoviolence, 1–2,